MENOPAUSE

THE ANSWERS

Understand and manage symptoms
with natural solutions, alternative remedies
and conventional medical advice

DR ROSEMARY LEONARD

First published in Great Britain in 2017
by Orion Spring
an imprint of The Orion Publishing Group Ltd
Carmelite House, 50 Victoria Embankment
London EC4Y 0DZ

An Hachette UK Company

1 3 5 7 9 10 8 6 4 2

A CIP catalogue record for this book
is available from the British Library.

ISBN: 978 1 4091 5334 4

Printed and bound by CPI Group (UK) Ltd, Croydon, CR0 4YY

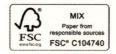

www.orionbooks.co.uk

ORION
SPRING

CONTENTS

INTRODUCTION

Hello.

I'm Dr Rosemary Leonard, and welcome to my guide to the menopause.

First, a bit about me. After I qualified as a doctor, I spent five years doing speciality training in obstetrics and gynaecology before I switched to general practice. I've always maintained a keen interest in women's health, and it seems I'm the go-to doctor in my area for women who want advice about the menopause – probably because it's something that I have experienced myself!

I'm now 60, and I had my 'here we go' moment around eight years ago when I suddenly found myself needing to shed my warm cardigan in the middle of a practice meeting on a cold winter's day. I thought I knew what to expect, but the dizzy spells and sudden irrational bouts of anxiety certainly took me by surprise. Overall, though, I don't think I had too bad a time, especially compared to some of my girlfriends or patients who would come to me in desperation, asking what on earth they could do to make life through the change more bearable.

But not all women have a rough time, and at the other end of the scale are those who breeze through the menopause with seemingly no problems at all, and never go to see a doctor. But there are many others who come to see me for advice, not because they are having terrible symptoms, but because they are aware that the menopause marks a time in life when you really do need to take steps to look after yourself if you want a long, healthy life for the 40 or so years after your periods stop.

The menopause is something that happens to every woman, usually around the age of 50, and, being honest, I haven't met many who are eager for it to happen. Yes, there are some who say they are really looking forward to the day when they don't have periods, but it's the rest of the stuff that goes with the menopause that so many women dread. Hot flushes, sweats, thinning hair – everywhere – and no sex drive. Not forgetting the fact that you really can't have any more children. OK, you may not want any more children, but as a woman I know that's very different from not being *able* to have any more children.

HOW TO USE THIS BOOK

This book is a manual to guide you through the years before, during and after the menopause; to explain why symptoms are occurring and, more importantly, what you can do about them.

THE question that women always ask me is: 'Do I need HRT?', so I've included a big section about that, as well as another on alternative remedies.

Then there is information on managing other problems that can occur, such as mood swings, changes in your skin and hair and dealing with contraception. And there's advice on controlling your waistline, which suddenly seems to have a mind of its own the moment you hit 50.

In each section you'll find the common questions that women ask me, then some real case histories (though the names have, of course, been changed).

I've aimed to make this a manual that you can dip in and out of – you don't have to read it cover to cover. So if you want information about a specific topic – for example, hot flushes, mood swings or trying to do something about your weight – you should be able to get useful information from just one chapter. Like any manual, you'll find cross-references throughout to other pages elsewhere in the book so that you can easily find more information if you need it.

What I'm aiming to do with this book is to give you the facts, so that you know what may be happening, or about to happen, and what you can do about it. I hope, too, that this gives you some down-to-earth advice about keeping fit and healthy right through the menopause, and into the years ahead.

BEING HEARD – GETTING THE BEST FROM YOUR DOCTOR

Throughout this book there will be times when I will direct you to get advice or further help from your GP. I'd be the first to admit that in the current cash-strapped NHS, this is easier said than done. Getting past the receptionist, let alone actually getting an appointment, can seem like climbing Everest. And then when you finally do get into the consulting room, you leave with a sense of being short-changed – that the doctor hadn't really got a clue about managing the menopause, or didn't have the time to listen to you and actually sort your symptoms out properly.

There is no magic solution to this, but here are some tips I can give you that might make it a bit easier for you to get a decent service from your surgery, and your GP.

Appointments

Rules set by the NHS mean that GPs have to offer a mix of appointments – some for advance booking, and some for booking on the day – which are usually split into morning and afternoon appointments. GPs are also encouraged to have appointments that can be booked online, and for menopause problems I'd recommend this route as it's easier than doing battle with the surgery phone system. You will need to get a login password from the surgery reception desk. Appointments for the same day are usually released around 8.30am and 2pm, but check with your individual surgery. There are also often appointments that are released a couple of days in advance, so it could be that you can't get an appointment with your favourite doctor when you ring on Monday, but you can get one for later in the week if you ring on Tuesday. If your doctor works part-time, it can help to find out from the receptionist the best time to ring to get an appointment with him or her.

And talking of favourite doctors ...

There is often a doctor in the practice, or one of the nurses, who has a special interest in women's health, and he or she will be more informed and up to date about menopause matters than the others. Find out who this is by asking at reception. In most practices it is perfectly acceptable to see a different GP for different problems.

But what if the receptionist is acting like a roadblock?

The most important thing here is to keep calm and to remember that they are just trying to do their job. There is a national shortage of GPs and there simply aren't enough appointments to meet the demand. Don't lose your temper, or be rude. Rather, be polite and honest and explain why you want an appointment. Far better to get a reputation as someone who is friendly than awkward – it can make a big difference.

What if the doctor seems rushed and keeps cutting me off mid-sentence?

The time when this is most likely to happen is if you are being long-winded about a problem or are telling the doctor stuff that is already written on your computer records that are in front of them. A standard GP appointment is only 10 minutes long, and often this really isn't enough (which is why surgeries often don't run to time). Try to keep your story, and symptoms, as concise as possible, and write a list if you think this would be helpful. Most importantly when it comes to menopausal issues, know the dates of your last few periods and how long they have lasted. It's amazing how many women who come to see me have to get their diaries out for this, which wastes valuable time.

Can I ask for a new treatment I've read about?

GPs have to do some training every year to keep up to date, but medicine is a fast-moving area and it can be difficult to keep abreast of every new development. So there's no harm in mentioning a new treatment that you have heard of, but be aware that some new medical developments that get publicity are either years away from being available to the public or as yet have no evidence at all for actually doing any good. So be prepared for your doctor to either say they need to do some of their own research, or to give you a firm 'no'.

What if I've got private insurance? Surely I can demand to see a specialist?

No, not really. The reason why insurers ask for a GP referral letter is to make sure that you do actually need to see a specialist (otherwise everyone's premiums would rise astronomically). Not only that, but even if you do get a letter, you will need to contact your insurer to have the costs of seeing a specialist authorised. Most insurers expect GPs to be able to manage menopause issues such as hot flushes, sweats, mood changes or heavy periods. You are only likely to be able to get your costs covered to see a specialist if you have an issue that has persisted despite treatment from your GP, such as very heavy periods that lead to anaemia, or when a pre-existing medical condition, such as breast cancer, makes treatment tricky.

1

THE MENOPAUSE
AND PERIMENOPAUSE

In this chapter I'm going to give you some basic information about the menopause, in particular why and when it happens. And in the second half of this chapter I will provide you with information about the perimenopause – the time of a woman's life that occurs in the run-up to the menopause itself.

I'll start with the questions that women most commonly ask me in my surgery.

SO, THE MENOPAUSE. WHAT IS IT?

The medical profession defines the menopause as the date of your last ever period. If only it was as simple as that!

The reality is that 'the menopause', like puberty, isn't a single event, it's something that happens gradually over a period of many months. And what is actually happening is that your ovaries are winding down and ceasing to produce both eggs and hormones. For some, the events surrounding the menopause can go on for years, and many women describe themselves during this time as being 'menopausal'. However, strictly speaking, according to gynaecologists, you can't be 'menopausal' while you are still having periods – even if they are all over the place. In this situation you are described as 'perimenopausal', which means you have not yet started the menopause.

Once your periods have stopped, according to doctors you are 'post-menopausal'. However, there is, of course, a grey area here, when you don't know whether your periods have finished or not.

How do I know if I'm menopausal?

The main sign of the menopause, which happens to every woman, is that their periods stop. Sometimes this happens suddenly; your cycle is pretty regular, then you don't have a bleed when you expect it and never have another one. But a much more common scenario is for periods to become very erratic and totally unpredictable. You may have a gap of six or eight weeks between two periods, then have three in a row, only a couple of weeks apart. This pattern may go on for six months or more – there's just no way of knowing when your periods are going to stop. A lot of women get other symptoms, too, such as hot flushes and sweats, as well as mood swings, but some very lucky women just realise their periods have come to an end. Nothing else. It's not necessarily a nightmare time for everyone.

What exactly is happening in my body?

What's actually happening is the ovaries have stopped working; they are no longer releasing eggs nor producing any hormones.

All women are born with a finite number of follicles in their ovaries, which each contain a tiny immature egg. Unlike men, who can continue to produce sperm until a ripe old age, women cannot produce any brand-new eggs at any time in their lives. The eggs that are released during her reproductive life are those that were there when she was born. At birth, a baby girl has around two million immature eggs in her ovaries, and from then on, they begin to shrink and disappear. By puberty, the number has dropped to around 400,000. Only around 500 follicles ever mature to develop and release an egg, the vast majority disappear of their own accord. The menopause marks the time when there are simply none left.

The most obvious result of this is that a woman can no longer conceive a baby. But the developing follicles are also the main source of hormones, which means that at the menopause their levels fall drastically.

The ovaries produce three main hormones – oestrogen, progesterone and also small amounts of testosterone. (There's more about this on page 236.) The sex hormones (as they are known) don't just act on the womb and the genital tissues, there are also receptors for these hormones in other parts of the body, including the breasts, bones, skin and connective tissue and brain. This means the hormones have a profound influence on a woman's life from puberty, when the ovaries start working, for the next 40 or so years, playing a major role not just in fertility but in physical and emotional wellbeing, too. So it's no wonder that when the ovaries stop working it can be a time of profound change for women.

It's the loss in oestrogen that causes most of the symptoms that occur during the menopause, especially flushes and sweats. In the following years, lack of oestrogen can lead to vaginal dryness, loss of sex drive, thinning of the bones (osteopenia and osteoporosis) and a general reduction in the supporting collagen in the skin and the genital area, leading to less fullness in the skin, more wrinkles and a tendency to incontinence. I'm aware that this sounds like a pretty awful list, but it's really not all doom and gloom, and there is plenty you can do to maintain both your appearance and your health for the many years that follow when you don't have oestrogen.

Is there a test to tell me when the menopause is going to occur?

The main test that is used to determine whether you are menopausal is the one that analyses your level of Follicle-stimulating Hormone, or FSH. This is the hormone that is produced by the pituitary gland that drives the ovaries. During the reproductive years, when the ovaries are working, FSH stimulates the ovaries to produce oestrogen, and when oestrogen reaches a threshold level, it is detected by the pituitary, which switches off, so FSH levels then fall. It's nature's way of keeping the whole system under control.

At the menopause, the fall in oestrogen means that the pituitary pours out more and more FSH to try to get the ovaries to keep working. So a rise in FSH can be used to detect when the ovaries are no longer working.

Unfortunately, doing the test is not straightforward. The ovaries don't stop working in a nice orderly way, but rather they will work well one day and not very well the next (this is one reason for the wild mood swings that some women get at this time in their life). This also means that FSH levels can vary enormously from one day to the next. My local laboratory grades an FSH up to 12 as being normal; between 13 and 25 as 'perimenopausal' and over 26 as menopausal, but I've seen plenty of women with an FSH in the high twenties and thirties one day and then when it's checked a month later it is down in the teens. I think measuring FSH levels is only useful to see if your ovaries have well and truly packed up, in which case the level will be over 100. But it's not much use in the perimenopause for trying to predict when your periods are going to stop and, in fact, this test is no longer officially recommended.

So when is it going to occur?

The average age of the menopause in women in the UK is 51, and most women have their last period between the ages of 49 and 53. However, it's considered normal for it to occur five years before or after this age, and there is nothing unusual about going through the menopause at 46 or 56.

Many women, especially those in their early forties who have not yet started a family, are keen to know how long their supply of follicles will last. If you only have a couple of years of fertility left, it's understandable to want to know about it! Unfortunately, predicting the age at which the menopause will occur is extremely difficult.

Is there anything I can do to change the timing of the menopause?

In the vast majority of women, the menopause will happen at a time decided by your own body, and there is nothing that you can do about it.

However, there are some factors that are known to play a role, and these are listed on page 13. The most important one that you can actually do something about is smoking – the more your ovaries have been exposed to cigarette smoke, the earlier they are likely to stop working.

SOME BACKGROUND BIOLOGY

The ovaries are two small structures, usually a bit smaller than a standard hen's egg, that sit in the middle pelvis on either side of the womb. The ovaries contain both glandular tissue and also numerous immature follicles, which each contain a tiny egg.

The ovaries produce three main hormones: the most important ones are oestrogen and progesterone, but in addition they produce small amounts of testosterone.

The control centre for the ovaries and the menstrual cycle is the pituitary gland, which is located in the base of the brain. The pituitary produces two hormones: Follicle-stimulating Hormone (FSH) and Luteinising Hormone (LH), and these in turn control the day-to-day workings of the ovaries.

To explain what happens to hormone levels during the menstrual cycle it's easiest to start with the first day of a period. Levels of FSH slowly begin to rise, and this stimulates the development of one of the immature follicles. As the follicle grows, the egg it contains slowly develops and grows, and the cells surrounding it produce increasing amounts of the most potent type of oestrogen, which is called oestradiol. Small amounts of oestrogen are also produced by the glandular tissue, but the vast majority comes from the developing follicle. The oestrogen stimulates the growth of the lining of the womb and also has actions elsewhere in the body. In the vagina, the amount of natural secretion also gradually increases in response to the rising oestrogen levels. When they peak, which occurs just before ovulation, some women notice this as a slightly sticky, clear discharge. It's nature's signal that you are at your most fertile.

In a typical monthly cycle, FSH and oestrogen levels carry on rising for the next 12 to 13 days. The pituitary gland detects when oestrogen rises above a threshold value and responds by producing a sudden surge of LH. This in turn triggers the release of the egg, which is now mature, from the follicle. This first or follicular phase of the menstrual cycle can be of a varying length. In most women it is around 12 to 14 days, in others it can be several weeks. It's the follicular phase that determines whether you have regular periods or not.

Following ovulation, the now-empty follicle, called a corpus luteum, produces the hormone progesterone. This acts on the womb lining, making the cells more mature. It's nature at work again, preparing the womb so it is ready for a potential fertilised egg.

Some oestrogen is also produced after ovulation, though in smaller amounts than in the first half of the cycle. Levels of both hormones continue to rise for about a week after ovulation, then they begin to fall (unless the egg is fertilised). The rich, thick womb lining is sustained by both hormones, but when levels fall low below a certain level, it becomes unstable and is shed as a period. Unlike the follicular phase, the time between ovulation and the start of a period, known as the luteal phase, is always the same length, about 14 days.

The third hormone that is produced by the ovaries is testosterone. Traditionally this is viewed as a male hormone, and it's true that levels found in men are vastly higher than those found in women, but the small amounts of testosterone that the ovaries produce play an important part in a woman's sex drive.

The ovarian tissue does continue to produce some oestrogen and testosterone after the menopause, and small amounts of a much weaker form of oestrogen – oestrone – are produced by fat cells. The adrenal glands also produce small amounts of testosterone, but overall the amounts are tiny compared to when the ovaries were working at their best.

More about the timing of the menopause

Unfortunately, most of the factors that govern the timing of the menopause are completely outside of your control – there is nothing you can do about them.

These include:

- The number of follicles you are born with is clearly the most important factor of all. This is impossible to measure, although maybe in the not-too-distant future a clever scientist somewhere will find a method of counting follicles in teenage girls. Having either an early or late menopause can run in families, so your genes can play a role. That said, just because your mother had a late menopause doesn't mean that you definitely will too – you just have an above-average chance of having a late menopause.

- Occasionally an early menopause can be linked with autoimmune disorders, particularly Type 1 diabetes and thyroid disease.

- Starting your periods at an early age, before 12 years old, can increase the risk of having a slightly earlier menopause. It would be easy to say this is because the eggs start being produced, and are used up, earlier, but this can't be the whole story. After all, only 12 eggs are used on average in a year by ovulation, and a lot more than that shrink of their own accord.

The one big factor that you do have control over which can influence the timing of the menopause is smoking. Smoking narrows the arteries, therefore reducing blood and oxygen supply to every tissue in the body. The ovaries aren't excluded from this, and women who smoke are likely to have a menopause two years earlier than non-smokers. There is also evidence that women exposed to secondhand smoke are more at risk of a slightly earlier menopause.

What about surgery?

There is evidence that women who have their womb removed (known as a hysterectomy) go through the menopause a couple of years earlier than average, even if their ovaries are left untouched by the surgery. It is thought that a slight disruption to the blood supply to the ovaries may be the cause of this.

Hysterectomy is a term that women often use to describe several different operations, although it actually means the removal of just the womb. If the ovaries are removed as well, this should be specified as 'a hysterectomy and oophorectomy'. Any woman who has had, or is about to have, a hysterectomy should make sure she knows what has happened to, or is planned for, her ovaries. Removing both ovaries produces a sudden menopause, but removing only one ovary should not have any effect – the other ovary just takes over from the missing one.

If a woman receives treatment for cancer, some chemotherapy drugs can kill off not just the cancerous cells but also the developing follicles in the ovaries, which can lead to a sudden loss of ovarian function.

THE PERIMENOPAUSE

'My cycle changed in my early forties. Instead of having a period every 29 days, they came every 25 days, but they were still quite regular. Then, suddenly, at the age of 49, I had a gap of six weeks, followed by the most horrendous heavy bleed. Thank goodness I was at home – for half an hour I sat on the loo and just bled. If I hadn't known it was impossible, I'd have thought I was having a miscarriage. I managed to get through the rest of the day by wearing a tampon and a large pad – no skinny jeans that day – and then mercifully the bleeding returned to a normal period for the next four days. I was really worried that it would happen again when I was at work, and after that I always carried extra protection in my handbag, plus a spare pair of knickers. My cycle returned to normal for the next three months, then the same thing happened again – this time after a gap of seven weeks. Luckily this time the bleeding wasn't quite so heavy. I also started getting the odd hot flush, but that didn't worry me nearly so much as the possibility of a heavy bleed when I was at work. My periods finally stopped a year after that first horrendous bleed. I'll always remember it – it was by far the worst thing about the perimenopause for me.'

'At the age of 50 my periods started going erratic, but though some were heavy, I could cope OK. It was more the tender breasts that bothered me. My breasts were so sore, all the time, as if I was premenstrual all the time. My doctor said it was because of the hormone imbalance that was going on – I wasn't ovulating so there was no progesterone to balance the effect of oestrogen on my boobs. I tried evening primrose oil, but as my doctor had warned me, it didn't do any good. The only answer was to wear a really supportive bra, all the time (including at night-time) and take paracetamol on the bad days. It went on for about four months, then my periods stopped and I could touch my chest again without wincing.'

'The first time I had a hot flush I thought I was going down with the flu. I was sitting at my desk at work and suddenly felt odd, really hot and sweaty. But then after a couple of minutes it passed. I was 49 at the time, and my periods were still regular, so it was a bit unexpected. After that I started getting flushes a few times a day, but generally they weren't too bad. My periods never went erratic – they just suddenly stopped four months after the flushes started, and the flushes stopped a few months after that. I made sure I could shed a layer if I needed to, and avoided wearing anything made out of polyester for a few months, as it made me feel a bit sticky when I was sweaty. But for me, the whole perimenopause thing really wasn't that bad. I certainly didn't need to take any pills or supplements.'

So what is the perimenopause?

The menopause does not happen suddenly. The functioning of the ovaries changes from the late thirties onwards. It's common for women in their early forties to notice that the gap between periods shortens by a few days, so that periods occur every 25 or 26 days, rather than every 28 days. However, this does *not* mean that the menopause is approaching and that you are perimenopausal. In fact, the perimenopause is the time when your ovaries are clearly not working as well as they were before.

This state of affairs can, and often does, continue for the next 10 years.

The signs that you could be in the perimenopause include:

- an erratic menstrual cycle, especially when previously your cycle has been regular

- missing periods

- hot flushes and sweats

- mood swings.

All of these – especially mood swings – can be due to other factors, but from the mid-forties onwards, a change in your ovarian function is top of the list of possible causes.

Is there a blood test that will show what's going on?

Unfortunately, testing to see if you are perimenopausal is not straightforward.

The ovaries do not wind down in a regular fashion, rather they will work well one day and not very well the next. This can lead to wild variations in hormone levels. The most common test used for checking menopause status is checking for blood levels of FSH. As oestrogen levels fall, the pituitary gland responds by producing more FSH, in an attempt to stimulate the ovaries into action. That means that FSH levels rise at the approach of the menopause. Measuring LH can be helpful, too.

According to most laboratories, an FSH level of 40IU/L or above means that you are post menopause. An FSH level of less than 11 is not suggestive of the menopause. Interpreting levels between 11 and 40 is more difficult; if the FSH level is less than the LH level, then a midcycle surge in hormones could be to blame, but if the FSH level is greater than 11 and less than the LH level, then the perimenopause might be to blame. This is more likely if the FSH level is above 27.

But it's no good relying on one test alone for diagnosing the perimenopause, because levels can vary not only from one day to the next, but from hour to hour. The best time to measure hormone levels is always during a period, particularly during the first few days, as this is when they are at their lowest, but even then the level may be higher at 10am than it is at 11am. In men, testosterone levels are predictably lowest first thing in the morning, but sadly the same rule does not apply to the sex hormones in women, and there is no way of predicting at which time of day oestrogen and FSH levels are going to be at their highest or lowest. So you could have a blood test done at noon on day three of your period and the FSH could be in the normal range, then have another taken at 9 o'clock the following day which could suggest you are in the menopause.

What this all means is that having just one blood test done is usually not very helpful, unless the FSH level is sky-high – by which I mean greater than 100IU/L. That sort of level is indicative that the ovaries have really stopped working and you are post menopause. But a woman in the perimenopause could have levels of 50IU/L one day and 13IU/L a couple of days later. So if you really want to know if you are approaching the menopause you need to have at least two blood tests done, at least a month apart. But even then, unless the levels are really high, they are not going to be much use in predicting when your periods are going to stop. In reality, the blood tests are only helpful if you want to know if you are still fertile – the higher the FSH level, the lower your fertility. But blood tests really don't make much difference to managing troublesome symptoms.

Why am I sometimes having horrendously heavy periods, especially when I've not had problems with my periods before?

As I've described above, during the perimenopause the ovaries work in a very erratic fashion. One day they can produce far more oestrogen than the next. Not only that, but the monthly release of an egg no longer occurs in a predictable way, so periods can become very erratic. One month you may release an egg and have a period at the usual, expected time. But the next month ovulation may not occur. This means that there is no progesterone to balance the effects of oestrogen; the womb lining carries on becoming thicker and thicker, until eventually, after about six weeks, it breaks down, causing an extremely heavy period. (There's much more about this in Chapter 7.)

The wild fluctuations in oestrogen levels can also lead to mood swings and tender breasts. No wonder some women in the perimenopause say they feel as if they have bad premenstrual syndrome all the time.

PREMATURE MENOPAUSE

'My periods went erratic when I was 38. To begin with I blamed stress – I was working full-time and had two kids under six and I was aware that I never had any time for myself. I also thought that was why I was always so tired. But then I started getting hot flushes and sweats, and that's when I went to see my doctor. I was worried I had a thyroid problem – the thought of the menopause at my age hadn't crossed my mind. But the blood tests showed it wasn't my thyroid that wasn't working, it was my ovaries. It was a complete shock, and really knocked me, mentally. My doctor gave me HRT, which stopped the flushes, but I didn't feel like a proper woman any more. My partner and I had decided that we didn't want any more children after our second one was born, but the fact I actually couldn't have any more was really horrible. I felt broody, and couldn't face looking at pregnant women for a long time. Five years on, I've come to terms with it and realise I'm actually one of the lucky ones – at least I'd already got children when it happened.'

Occasionally the menopause can occur before the age of 40. Medically termed 'Premature Ovarian Insufficiency' (POI), this affects about one in 100 women, and can occur in women in their teens or twenties, though it is more common in women in their thirties.

Why me?

Often the reason is not clear, but it is thought to be caused by either having a reduced number of follicles at birth or an accelerated loss of follicles. In some women it is an autoimmune condition, where antibodies develop against the ovarian tissue. It can occasionally also occur as a result of infectious diseases affecting the ovaries, such as mumps or tuberculosis (TB).

The first symptoms of POI are often erratic periods and sometimes hot flushes and sweats. Some women only discover their ovaries have seemingly stopped working when they have tests done to find out why they are failing to get pregnant.

Does that mean I can't get pregnant?

It depends on the underlying cause. If there are no follicles left, the situation is just like the menopause at a later age and a pregnancy cannot occur. However, if the problem is autoimmune, where the ovaries do contain follicles but are not working because of antibodies against the ovarian tissue, sometimes the antibody levels fluctuate and the ovaries spontaneously start working again. This means that pregnancies can, and do, occur, and I have seen women with POI being very surprised when they become pregnant. This is more likely to occur in the first few years of the condition.

So why was I having periods when I was on the Pill? Were my ovaries working then?

The combined contraceptive pill stops the ovaries working – which is why it is so good at preventing a pregnancy! It contains oestrogen and progesterone, so you don't notice you are not producing any naturally yourself, and the monthly 'period' is actually a withdrawal bleed, which occurs when you stop taking the hormones for a week each month. So it is often the case that women only realise they have had a premature menopause when they stop taking the Pill and their periods don't restart. I should add here, though, that premature menopause is a rare cause of this occurring – other problems, such as polycystic ovary syndrome (PCOS), are much more likely to be to blame.

So is there any way of knowing how long my ovaries are going to keep working?

Many women in their late thirties, who have delayed starting a family, are concerned about how long their ovaries will continue to function. Though it's currently not possible to predict exactly when the menopause will occur, the best test available at the moment is to measure the level of Anti-Mullerian Hormone (AMH). This is a protein produced by the growing follicles inside the ovaries, and can be detected in women from birth to near the menopause, with a peak in the mid-twenties. Levels of AMH fall steadily from the age of 25 onwards, and the lower the level, the smaller the 'ovarian reserve' or functioning ovarian tissue. Unlike levels of FSH, which change throughout the menstrual cycle, AMH levels stay fairly constant, so can be measured at any time. AMH is used mainly as a predictor for how successful fertility treatment is likely to be, as those with high levels of this hormone are more likely to respond to drugs that stimulate ovulation compared to those with low levels of it. AMH is not used as a diagnostic test for the menopause, as levels are usually low from the mid-forties onwards. However, for women in their thirties it can be used as a predictor for whether or not they are likely to have an early menopause – the higher the level, the longer the ovaries are likely to keep working.

Is there any test for premature menopause?

In younger women, checking the FSH level can be helpful, though it can vary a bit from day to day. If the ovaries are functioning normally, the level should be 12 or below; a level higher than this makes a premature menopause a likely diagnosis, though it's wise to do a second test at least a week later. It's also possible to do a blood test for ovarian antibodies. Though a negative test doesn't rule out a premature menopause, a positive test makes the diagnosis more likely.

Melinda, age 48

HER STORY: My periods were regular until a couple of months ago, but now I've just missed one – there was a gap of eight weeks between my last one and the one that's just started now. Does this mean I'm menopausal? If so, when are the flushes going to start? And what exactly is happening in my body? Is there a test you can do that will tell me for sure when my periods are going to stop?

MY ADVICE: The change in her periods suggested that she was approaching the menopause. However, I had to tell her that there wasn't a test she could do that would say when her periods were going to stop. Checking her FSH levels wouldn't help – even if the level was very high today, it could be lower the next day and it wouldn't tell her if she was going to have another period. Similarly, there is no way of knowing if she was going to have hot flushes or not – she will just have to wait and see what happens!

Angie, age 46

HER STORY: My periods have always been a bit erratic. My last one was four months ago, but this has happened before. I'm not having flushes or sweats, but I'm aware I'm quite moody, and I often get really anxious about silly little things, which isn't like me at all. I am under stress at work, but I wondered if it's the menopause? Is there any way of finding out?

MY ADVICE: It would have been possible to do a check of her FSH levels, but it was unlikely to be very helpful, unless it was sky-high, indicating that her ovaries had stopped working completely. Not only that, but it wouldn't be very helpful in managing her symptoms. It was the mood swings and anxiety that were bothering her, and although if she was menopausal HRT might help a bit, there are better, non-hormonal treatments for this type of problem, such as cognitive behavioural therapy, or antidepressants. (There is more information about this in Chapter 2.)

Flo, age 43

HER STORY: My cycle has changed. I always used to have periods every 29 days, counting between the first day of one and the first day of the next. But for the last five months they are coming more frequently, every 25 days, though they are still regular. I haven't got any other symptoms, like hot flushes, but does this change in my cycle mean I'm perimenopausal? And if so, how long before my periods stop altogether?

MY ADVICE: It was very unlikely that Flo was in the perimenopause. She still had a regular cycle, indicating that her ovaries were working normally. Her shortened cycle was normal for a woman in her early forties, and was not in any way a sign that her periods were about to stop altogether. When that will happen is impossible to predict, but as with most women, it's likely that her periods will stop somewhere around the age of 51.

Kate, age 49

HER STORY: For the last few months my periods have been really erratic and completely unpredictable. One month I had two, then I had a six-week gap before I had a horrendously heavy one. And I've noticed I'm getting a bit more moody. I presume this means I'm perimenopausal, but how long is this going to carry on? Is there a test you can do which can show you when my periods are going to stop?

MY ADVICE: The pattern of erratic periods at her age suggests that she was approaching the menopause. Unfortunately, there isn't a test that can show when periods are going to stop. Checking the level of FSH – which 'drives' the ovaries – is hopelessly unreliable, it might suggest her ovaries were working normally one day, and then the next if checked again it could suggest she was menopausal. It's impossible to know how long this completely erratic pattern of bleeding will continue, but in my experience it's unusual for 'menstrual chaos' to last more than a year. But if the bleeding really became a nuisance, I advised her that there are treatments that can help.

Janey, age 48

HER STORY: I'm not sure what is happening with my periods. I still seem to get what I'd call a 'normal' period every month, but I'm getting some bleeding in between them as well. It's generally a bit lighter than a period, sometimes just a bit of spotting. This tends to happen especially after sex. Does this mean I'm perimenopausal? I do feel a bit anxious sometimes, but haven't had any flushes or sweats.

MY ADVICE: Though erratic bleeding can be a sign of the perimenopause, it is very unusual for hormone changes alone to cause spotting between periods, or after sex. This type of bleeding is much more likely to be due to another cause, unrelated to hormones, such as a small polyp (or outgrowth) from the lining of the womb or cervix, or an infection. When I examined her I could see nothing unusual, but an ultrasound scan showed she had a small polyp extending from the lining of her womb into her cervix, which was the cause of her bleeding. It was removed during a small operation, and after that her unusual bleeding stopped.

Rose, age 34

HER STORY: I came off the Pill a year ago, because my partner and I wanted to start a family. Since then I haven't had a period. I've done loads of pregnancy tests and they have all been negative. But what's worrying me now is I'm having hot flushes and sweats. A friend suggested it could be the menopause, but I'm far too young for that, surely?

MY ADVICE: The combination of no periods, flushes and sweats does suggest the possibility of the menopause, which occasionally does happen in young women. I suggested we do a blood test for her FSH level, and also for ovarian antibodies. Her FSH was 34, suggesting that her ovaries were not working properly, which was due to her high level of ovarian antibodies. She was understandably devastated, especially as she wanted a baby. After I had given her some time for the news to sink in, I suggested she have HRT, to help stop her flushes and sweats, to protect her bones, and also to help maintain her skin and hair. I told her that the dose of oestrogen was low, and that it would not stop her ovulating if her ovaries did start working again.

She gradually seemed to come to terms with her fate, and started thinking about adoption. However, two years later, she came to see me because she had not had her usual monthly HRT withdrawal bleed and, rather miraculously, she was pregnant. She went on to have a healthy baby boy. After her pregnancy, she immediately became menopausal again, and only had the one child.

SUMMARY

- 📖 The menopause marks the time when a woman's ovaries stop working. They no longer produce any eggs, periods stop and a woman's fertile years are at an end. They also stop producing hormones, and the dramatic decline in oestrogen in particular can lead to flushes, sweats and mood swings.

- 📖 The average age at which the menopause occurs is 51, but it's normal for it to happen five years on either side of this. Occasionally the menopause occurs before the age of 46, in which case it's known as a premature menopause. Occasionally it can occur at a much earlier age, often because the body's immune system develops antibodies that attack ovarian tissue.

- 📖 The ovaries may work in a very erratic way in the run-up to the menopause, causing erratic and sometimes heavy periods, often with really bad accompanying premenstrual syndrome (PMS). This time is known as the perimenopause, but it rarely lasts more than a couple of years.

- 📖 It's normal for the menstrual cycle to become a little shorter after a woman has turned 40, with periods occurring every 26 days instead of 28. This change does not signify you are approaching the menopause.

- 📖 Testing to see if you are in the perimenopause can be very difficult, as the ovaries work so erratically and hormone levels change from day to day.

- 📖 There is no accurate way of predicting when you are going to become menopausal, though some factors – such as smoking, a family history of an earlier menopause, or having your womb removed – can mean you are slightly more likely to have an earlier menopause than the average woman.

2

....

THE DREADED FLUSHES AND SWEATS

There are some lucky women who go through the menopause without ever having a flush or producing an extra bead of sweat, but they are in the minority. Others find their life is made a complete misery by their body thermostat seeming to be completely out of control – feeling hot and dripping in sweat one minute, then freezing cold the next.

I was one of the many who were somewhere between these two extremes. I remember sitting in a car on the way back from the BBC and for the whole of the journey I was constantly taking my jacket off, then putting it on again, opening the window, then closing it. And I also felt a bit nauseous – something that a lot of women only mention when asked about it. But that type of episode didn't happen often, and I didn't have too many sleepless nights.

What I'm going to do in this chapter is explain when flushes and sweats might occur, and how long you can expect them to continue. This chapter also includes information on the lifestyle changes that can ease flushes and sweats, as well as non-hormonal medications that can help. There's also a big section on 'alternative' remedies.

The key questions that women want answered:

Flushes and sweats. I keep hearing about them, but what exactly are they?

Flushes are usually experienced as an uncomfortable hot sensation that starts in the chest and works up to the face. These can last anything from a few minutes to, if you're really unlucky, half an hour. This sensation may, or may not, be accompanied by beads of perspiration appearing most commonly on your forehead and also your hands. But worse sweating can occur, where you feel a bit damp all over. This tends to happen more at night. Thankfully, having horrific-looking wet patches on your clothes around your armpits (we've all seen this on the shirts of hot sweaty men) is actually very rare.

Are they two different things? Is it possible to get flushes without sweats, and vice versa, or do you always get both?

Both flushes and sweats are caused by the fall in oestrogen levels that occurs around the time of the menopause. They are often spoken of as if they occur together, but this isn't always the case. Some women get flushes but don't sweat, while others have bad sweats but don't have any flushing. And like other menopause symptoms, there's no way of predicting if you are going to get both – you just have to wait and see what happens.

Why do they happen?

It's the falling levels of oestrogen that occur at the time of menopause that are to blame. Changes in oestrogen levels can trigger a chain of events inside the brain, involving the chemicals serotonin and noradrenaline, that cause disruption to the working of the bit that controls your body temperature. It overreacts to just the weeniest change in temperature, and that, in turn, leads to flushes and sweats.

The exact reason why some women get terrible flushes and others get none at all isn't known – after all, every woman has a decline in her oestrogen levels at the time of the menopause. It is probably linked to genetic differences, and this probably also explains why the severity of flushes differs between women of different races and ethnicities.

Do I look as hot as I feel?

The good news is that you rarely look as hot as you feel. Many women are concerned that when they are having a hot flush their face must resemble a beetroot, but often the only outward sign is just slight blushing. And what may feel like a soaking sweat to you may be barely noticeable to anyone else. What makes a hot flush far more obvious is getting a fan out, or wiping your brow. If you just somehow ignore how you feel, the chances are no one else will have a clue what is going on. But that's easier said than done!

When do flushes and sweats start? How long are they going to carry on for?

In most women, flushes and sweats usually start when your menstrual cycle goes truly haywire. Others find that the flushes start around six months after their periods have stopped. It is unusual for them to start more than a year after your last period, though this does occasionally happen.

Unfortunately, it is incredibly difficult to say how long flushes and sweats are going to continue for. The generally accepted view is that in most women, flushes last six months to two years, but it can be much longer than this.

What can I do about them?

Each case has to be tackled individually, according to how much the sensations are affecting your quality of life. If the flushes and sweats are not too bad, making a few lifestyle adjustments may be enough to see you through the worst. But if you constantly feel like you are glowing like a beacon and nothing you do seems to help, taking medication to make life more bearable seems sensible.

Do I need HRT?

There is no doubt that HRT is the best treatment for flushes and sweats and can get rid of them within days, but whether you need it or not depends on lots of factors. Of prime importance is how much you are suffering and whether you are prepared to accept the risks and side effects associated with HRT. I think it's always worth trying other things first – such as lifestyle changes and maybe herbal remedies or supplements (see page 46), but if flushes and sweats continue to make your life a misery, HRT is the answer, unless there are medical reasons why you should not have it. HRT is also a very good option if you are having a rotten time with menopausal symptoms and are at high risk of osteoporosis. There is more information about this on page 65.

What if I don't want HRT? What are the alternatives? Do they work?

There are alternative drug treatments for flushes and sweats and they can be very helpful – though they are generally not as effective as HRT. The most commonly used ones are antidepressants (yes, you did read that correctly) and clonidine. There is more information about these on page 39.

Alternative remedies can also take the edge off symptoms in some women, and for more information about these, see pages 39–44.

Lifestyle changes can make a difference, too. I'll get on to these in the next section.

BACKGROUND BIOLOGY

This is for those of you who want the science. Skip it if you want, I've summarised it all more simply on page 26.

Rather strangely, for something that happens to so many people, the exact reason why hot flushes occur is not known. Lots of research has been done and is ongoing, and our knowledge base is certainly increasing, but there is still a lot we don't know.

If you look at a thermal-imaging picture of the skin during a hot flush it's possible to see the skin areas that feel hot (typically the face, neck and fingers) and then watch them as they cool down. This change in temperature is brought about by the widening, or 'vasodilation', of the tiny arteries within the skin, and the increase in heat that this produces also triggers sweating. But the fundamental question is why do these tiny arteries suddenly dilate with no change in outside temperature?

The temperature of our body is controlled by a thermoregulatory centre in the brain. This can respond to changes in the body's core temperature, triggering the mechanisms that produce shivering if the body becomes cold, or sweating if the body becomes too hot. Though this brain centre is incredibly sensitive, there is a small zone, called the 'null zone', which is thought to be about 0.4 degrees centigrade, where the body's temperature can fluctuate with no response. This is the body's way of not making you shiver or sweat at the weeniest change in temperature. It's thought that during hot flushes this thermoregulatory centre is disrupted, with even small changes eliciting an exaggerated response from the brain's control centre. In other words, the null zone no longer works.

Like so many other parts of the brain, the function of the temperature regulatory zone is influenced by several chemicals that can control brain cell function, including serotonin and noradrenaline.

These names may be familiar to you for another reason, as they are also the chemicals that are intricately involved in controlling your mood. Low levels of serotonin activity in particular are linked with depression.

It is now thought that oestrogen doesn't work directly on the thermoregulatory centre, but rather influences the levels of these neurotransmitter chemicals. It's not possible to measure brain serotonin levels in the general population – you can't do it with a blood test – but in research trials in post-menopausal women using functional MRI (magnetic resonance imaging) brain scanners, serotonin activity was boosted by giving hormone replacement therapy containing oestrogen. Similarly, drugs that block noradrenaline activity can trigger hot flushes, whereas those that increase noradrenaline, such as clonidine, can help decrease the occurrence of hot flushes.

But it's not just oestrogen that can affect serotonin and noradrenaline levels in the thermoregulatory zone. Both exercise and glucose have been shown to have a role, too.

The fact that the flushes are linked with changes in brain levels of serotonin and noradrenaline activity has opened up a whole new range of options for treating hot flushes, notably antidepressants, which alter the levels of these two chemicals in the brain. One thing to mention here is that these treatments seem to work by adjusting the thermoregulatory centre in the brain; they will only be effective as long as you take them, but it may well be that if you stop them after six months, then the worst will be over. Unlike HRT, there should be no rebound effect (see page 40) when you stop taking them, and again, unlike HRT, there are no long-term health risks associated with long-term use. Antidepressants can also be taken by the unlucky older women, in their sixties and seventies, who are continuing to get flushes and sweats.

If this sounds unlikely, it is true for some. I have personally come across many women who continue to have flushes well into their sixties. By this time oestrogen levels are stabilised at a low level, so it can't be fluctuating hormone levels that are to blame. It's more likely that there is a fundamental change in the functioning of the thermoregulatory centre instead. This would also explain why many post-menopausal women, though not suffering from flushes, say they sweat more easily than before, for example, when they are exercising, or that they generally feel less cold.

Unfortunately, there is no way of predicting how long flushes will last, or how bad they will be, in an individual woman. It remains an enigma as to why some women's bodies and thermoregulatory centres seem to adapt while others continue having flushes for a decade or more.

Some interesting research

A study done by the University of Philadelphia, published in 2011, monitored more than 300 women as part of an 'ovarian ageing' study. They found that the average length of hot flushes was 10 years. Interestingly, the commonest time for flushes to start was between the ages of 45 and 49, well before the menopause. Those who started flushes early were likely to have them for the longest period of time, while those that started them later, around the time of their last period, only had them on average for three years. There were also marked racial differences, with Afro-American women having flushes for longer than Caucasian women, and women with a high Body Mass Index (or BMI – see page 141) having more severe flushes than those who were slimmer. Though this study has been criticised for possible over-reporting of hot flushes, I have used it because there are several others that highlight the same findings. Flushes can, and often do, start well before periods start to become irregular, and may continue for years afterwards. And the fatter you are, the worse they are likely to be.

TACKLING FLUSHES AND SWEATS

Taking action to try to reduce flushes and sweats can be broadly divided into two groups – lifestyle changes, and taking tablets of some sort, either conventional medicine, or herbal supplements.

Clothing

- Wearing several layers of lighter clothing, rather than one thick layer, can be very helpful. When you feel hot, just shed a layer then put it back on again when you cool down.

- Get to know your clothing fibres and read labels carefully. Those items made from natural fibres are much better at allowing sweat to evaporate than man-made ones such as polyester. A blouse made with 45 per cent polyester and 55 per cent cotton can make you feel clammy and sticky as soon as you begin to sweat, but if you're wearing one made from 100 per cent cotton, you'll still feel fairly cool. In the hot summer months linen is a good choice, as long as you don't mind the creases!

- Viscose (also known as rayon) is also a natural fibre, but it's more moisture-absorbent than cotton, and breathable. So it is a good choice. However, like linen, it is prone to wrinkling.

- Acrylic, which is often used to make sweaters, can feel comfortable next to your skin, but it can make you more sweaty than fine wool. If you need the warmth of wool on a cold winter's day, wear something made of cotton as an underlayer – a T-shirt will do – which will feel much more comfortable when a hot moment strikes.

- Switch to bed linen made of 100 per cent cotton rather than a polycotton mix. I know it's much more of a faff to wash – it takes longer to dry and can look crumpled unless you have the time to run an iron over it – but it really can make a big difference to night-time comfort.

- The same goes for nightwear – switch to 100 per cent cotton.

- If you find yourself constantly throwing off the duvet, switch to one with a lower tog value. It may sound daft using a summer-weight, 4.5-tog duvet in the middle of winter, but it may be all you need. If necessary, add a blanket for extra warmth that you can throw off when heat strikes. Having two single duvets, of different weights, rather than a double, can solve the problem of your partner requiring a warmer duvet.

MY VERDICT: Always worth a try. These changes can definitely make life more bearable and take the edge off symptoms. But, being honest, they won't be enough if you are having really awful flushes and sweats.

Smoking

There have been several studies that suggest that smoking increases the risk of having bothersome, frequent hot flushes. The reason why this happens isn't known, but it may be because smoking alters the way oestrogen is metabolised in the body.

MY VERDICT: Smoking is so bad for your general health anyway, this is just another reason to give it up.

Being overweight

There is growing evidence that women who are overweight, and particularly those that are obese (with a Body Mass Index of 30 or more) are more prone to hot flushes. This may simply be because the excess fat acts as an insulating layer, but it may also be that chemicals produced by fat tissue interfere with temperature regulation in the body.

MY VERDICT: Like smoking, being obese is not good for your general health, so if you are having awful hot flushes, it's another stimulus to shed those excess pounds.

Exercise

Some women report that even moderate exercise makes hot flushes worse, and certainly it can make a tendency to sweat greater. However, a study in 2012 showed that immediately after a 30-minute session of moderate-intensity exercise, a significant number of the 92 women taking part reported fewer hot flushes, and this correlated with the monitors they were wearing to check their body temperature. The study also showed that women who were not physically fit before taking part in the study reported more hot flushes on the days that they did exercise.

In other words, exercise is likely to help your flushes if you are already fit, but make them worse to begin with if you've previously been a couch potato.

That said, exercise has so many other benefits for both peri- and post-menopausal women (weight management, increasing bone and muscle strength, boosting mood) that I think it should be top of every woman's priority list at the time of the menopause. Start gently with, for example, a brisk walk, or a swim, ideally at least twice a week, and gradually increase what you do. I know it can be difficult to find the time, but the more you do, the more you will benefit, the fitter you will become, and you should be less bothered by flushes and sweats.

However, it's best not to exercise just before you go to bed, as you are likely not only to feel warm afterwards, but more energised, which can disrupt sleep. Allow at least an hour of wind-down time afterwards before hitting the pillow.

MY VERDICT: It's good for you, and for getting rid of flushes and sweats, as long as you start gently if you've always been a couch potato. Make the time, and give it a go.

Yoga, relaxation techniques and paced respiration

Yoga has been shown to help lots of medical conditions, including anxiety and depression, but unfortunately well-designed studies have failed to show it is effective in alleviating hot flushes. That doesn't mean you should avoid it, but don't expect it to work miracles when you are feeling uncomfortable and sweaty.

MY VERDICT: Yoga is probably better for your muscles than for menopausal flushes.

Relaxation training includes methods such as special relaxation classes and relaxation tapes that you can use at home. The research that has been done on this so far suggests that it may help reduce hot flushes and sweats.

MY VERDICT: Worth a try if you have the time.

Paced respiration is a method of breathing that many women find useful when a hot flush is occurring. It involves taking slow, deep breaths, using your abdominal muscles, breathing in through your nose and out through your mouth. Breathe only five to seven times a minute – which is much slower than normal breathing. At first it may be obvious that you are breathing a little strangely, but with practice it usually becomes unnoticeable. Though there is no research evidence confirming its usefulness in alleviating hot flushes, there are anecdotal reports that some women find it helpful.

MY VERDICT: It's unlikely to do you any harm, so my view again is that it's worth a try if you've got the time. But if your time is limited, use it for proper exercise rather than paced respiration.

Diet

Making changes to your diet can help to reduce flushes and sweats, though the effects vary between women. If you are having really bad symptoms you may not notice much difference. But it is worth a try, and if you are only having occasional mild symptoms, this might be all you need to do to bring your life back to normal.

- Alcohol and caffeine can cause vasodilation (the medical term for the widening of arteries), and can make flushes and sweats worse. You are also likely to look more flushed. Don't stop drinking coffee suddenly, as this can cause awful caffeine-withdrawal headaches. Instead, cut down slowly and gradually switch to decaff.

- Eating really hot or spicy food can make anyone sweat, and can be a good way of triggering a really bad hot flush. Stick to mild kormas if you are having a curry, and let food cool a little on your plate before eating.

- Phytoestrogens are chemicals found naturally in plants that have a very weak oestrogen-like action. They work by stimulating oestrogen receptors throughout the body, but are only 1/1000 times as strong as the body's own oestrogen. However, it does seem that eating a diet rich in isoflavones can take the edge off hot flushes in some women.

MY VERDICT: Easy to do, and worth a try, but don't spend a fortune on special foods if you're not sure they are making any difference.

You can boost your phytoestrogen intake by eating more pulses, such as chickpeas and lentils, as well as beansprouts, linseeds, green leafy vegetables and especially soya products, such as tofu and soya milk. It's believed that 60 grams of natural soya product is enough to give a phytoestrogen effect. It's not a miracle remedy that's going to stop flushes and sweats, and neither is eating a plate of lentils going to stop a hot flush in its tracks, but it might just make flushes less severe, and adding natural phytoestrogen to your diet is very unlikely to do you any harm.

Soya has little flavour on its own but takes on the taste of the ingredients it is cooked with, so if you replace half the mince in a cooked dish – say a Bolognese sauce, with soya mince, it's unlikely that anyone will notice. It is also cheaper and lower in fat, too. You can add linseeds to lots of dishes, too.

As a last resort, a wide variety of supplements containing phytoestrogens are now available – see page 46.

Non-hormonal medication

The good news is that if flushes and sweats are making your life a misery, and you don't want to take HRT, there are several other treatments that have been proven to be helpful.

Antidepressants

Prescribing antidepressants is a relatively new approach to treating flushes and sweats, but it is one that is becoming increasingly popular. This is because not only do these drugs tackle suddenly feeling hot, but they can also help to reduce the mood changes that are so common at this time of life.

How do they work?

Most antidepressants have an effect on boosting the levels of either the brain chemicals serotonin or noradrenaline, or both. These chemicals are involved in controlling mood, but they also have an effect on the functioning of the body thermostat in the brain. This means that they not only help boost low mood, but they can also help to reduce flushes and sweats.

How quickly do they have an effect?

Unlike the antidepressant effect, which can take a week or more to really kick in, the drugs start to have an impact on the reduction in flushes and sweats within days of starting them.

Are there any side effects?

Yes, being honest these can be a problem, especially in the first few days. The main ones are a slight nausea, a dry mouth, and disturbed sleep, along with a slight increase in anxiety. But if you can get through the first few days, these symptoms usually lessen significantly.

Are the drugs addictive?

Antidepressants aren't addictive. The effects are so subtle that there is no urge to take another dose. However, stopping them suddenly can cause dizziness and headaches, so it's always wise to taper the dose down slowly when you decide you don't want to take them any more.

So is there a choice? Which one is best?

There are two main groups of antidepressants that can be used – Selective Serotonin Reuptake Inhibitors (SSRIs) and Serotonin and Noradrenaline Reuptake Inhibitors (SNRIs).

SSRIs include citalopram, escitalopram, sertraline and fluoxetine. Some studies have shown these to be 25 per cent more effective than placebo (dummy) pills at reducing the severity and number of hot flushes and sweats. The dosages that are effective for hot flushes are generally at the lower end of those used to treat depression.

The most commonly used SSRIs for menopausal symptoms are fluoxetine and citalopram. Citalopram has the advantage that it comes in a low dose – 10mg – as well as the standard 20mg, while fluoxetine only comes in a 20mg dose. This means that if you are concerned about side effects, citalopram is a good choice, starting with the low dose.

The most commonly used SNRI for flushes is venlafaxine, and this too comes in a low dose, 37.5mg, though the larger 75mg seems to be more effective for treating flushes and sweats.

Venlafaxine also seems to be more effective than SSRIs for menopausal symptoms, but its side effects can be more of a problem, and it's also more expensive, so doctors may be reluctant to prescribe it. It is also not suitable for women who have had heart disease or high blood pressure, and any woman taking venlafaxine should have her blood pressure checked every three months.

How long can I take them for?

There are no long-term health risks in taking these drugs, and many people are on them long term for depression. However, it does seem that their effect on treating flushes and sweats wears off after about nine months, but by this time, with luck, you should be over the worst of them anyway. And unlike stopping HRT, the symptoms won't suddenly rebound back when you do stop the drugs.

MY VERDICT: Definitely worth a try, especially if you are having troublesome moods swings or anxiety.

Harriet, age 57

'I kept sweating, especially at night, and because of that my sleep was really being disturbed. Switching to a lighter duvet didn't help – I just got cold! I tried eating extra soya, but it didn't seem to make any difference. I didn't want to take HRT because my mother had breast cancer. I'd read that exercise could help, but I don't know if it did or didn't for me, as I kept on sweating regardless of how much running I did. I was trying to avoid going to the doctor, as I thought I could manage the symptoms myself, but in the end I got so tired, I made an appointment. I was really surprised when she suggested antidepressants, as I didn't have any symptoms of depression. But she explained the science behind using them for menopausal symptoms, and I was so desperate I thought I'd give them a try, and chose fluoxetine. For the first few days I felt a bit odd – a bit anxious and nauseous – but after about a week the sweats did seem a bit better, and my sleeping definitely improved, though I did have some pretty weird dreams. After six months the sweats seemed to have gone – I don't know whether that was just nature taking its course or the pills, but I decided to come off the tablets. My doctor advised me to do this slowly, so I gradually reduced the dose and came off them over a period of six weeks. I've had the odd flush and sweat since then, but my sleeping is fine.'

More detailed background information

Many of the studies on these drugs have been done on women who have had breast cancer and who are therefore unable to take standard HRT, which contains oestrogen.

The most widely studied SNRI is venlafaxine, which in one study of 191 breast cancer survivors reduced flushes and sweats by 61 per cent, and in another trial of 80 women who had not had cancer, there was a significant difference in the reduction of hot flushes between those taking venlafaxine and those taking placebo pills. The best dose for reducing flushes and sweats appears to be 75mg a day, but because of side effects it is best to start with the lower dose of 37.5mg and gradually work up to 75mg.

Mirtazapine is a different kind of antidepressant (an NaSSA) that acts on both noradrenaline and serotonin levels in the brain. So far only small trials have been done, and though it does seem to show some benefits in reducing flushes and sweats, it causes a lot of sleepiness, and many of those in the trials stopped using it because of this. More research needs to be done to determine the best dose for reducing flushes while also minimising troublesome side effects.

And if antidepressants don't work, or cause too many side effects, is there anything else?

Gabapentin is used mainly as a treatment for seizures and also for chronic pain. Research has suggested that it can help reduce flushes and sweats, but only at higher doses (2400mg a day or more) which are more likely to cause side effects, such as dizziness and excessive sleepiness. It can also cause skin rashes, but all of these – if you can tolerate them – tend to improve over time. It can also cause puffiness of the feet and ankles, and weight gain, but not in everyone.

MY VERDICT: Maybe one to try if nothing else suits you or has worked.

Clonidine was originally developed as a treatment for high blood pressure but has also been used for many years to treat hot flushes. Traditionally only a very low dose of 25mcg daily is used, but this is rarely enough to be effective. Most women need at least 75mcg twice a day, and some double this. Side effects can include a dry mouth, dizziness, constipation and difficulty sleeping, and, of course, the higher the dose, the more likely these are to occur.

MY VERDICT: The dose required to be effective can cause really troublesome side effects. Another to try only if nothing else is suitable. If it hasn't helped after four weeks, there is little point in continuing it.

Helen, age 53

'I was getting quite bad flushes and sweats, but didn't want HRT – I just didn't like the sound of it. So I went to my GP to ask about alternatives. I certainly didn't want antidepressants either, so he gave me a prescription for gabapentin. But when I read the patient information leaflet, and all the possible side effects, I was really put off them. I confess I didn't even give them a try, but instead went back to the doctor. He suggested clonidine, which didn't sound quite so drastic as the other tablets. He gave me a tiny dose, and my flushes and sweats did get a bit better. Looking back, I don't know if that was the pills, or whether they would have got better anyway, but at least I didn't have any nasty side effects!'

Just to warn you, the drugs I've mentioned here have been around for many years, but their use in treating menopausal symptoms is fairly new. It's quite possible that your GP – who you'll need to see to get them prescribed for you – may never have heard of them being used in this way. In their defence, medicine is moving fast in lots of fields, and I know only too well that it can be difficult to keep up with everything, so if your GP looks at you blankly, take this book along with you!

Alternative Remedies

'I'm having a bad time with flushes and sweats. I don't want HRT, and the other medicines available on prescription that you've mentioned all seem to have scary sounding side effects. Are there any other options? What about alternative remedies, like herbal medicines?'

Go into any chemist or health-food shop and you'll find row upon row of remedies aimed at relieving symptoms of the menopause.

Many women consider HRT or antidepressants to be 'stronger' than they need – rather like the equivalent of taking a sledgehammer to try to crack a nut. Menopausal symptoms can make your life a bit of a misery, so it's no wonder that many women want to try something 'milder', as many of my patients put it. Something that will take the edge off the symptoms, but with no nasty side effects.

But unfortunately there are lots of unanswered questions about alternative remedies. Just because something is deemed to be 'natural', because it comes from plants, does not mean it is safe. After all, there are plenty of very powerful 'conventional' medicines that come from plants, such as digoxin, from foxgloves; atropine, from deadly nightshade; or Taxol, the chemotherapy agent that comes from yew trees.

Not only that, but there is a lack of conclusive scientific evidence that a number of them really do any good.

So what I'll try to do in this section is give some more background information about each product, what it claims to do, any side effects they may cause, and give my opinion on them.

More background information on the lack of research

One of the big problems with alternative remedies is the lack of really good research data. It is known that the 'placebo effect' can be very powerful – symptoms improve with dummy pills because the patient believes they are taking something that is beneficial. Research has shown that dummy pills can also cause side effects such as headaches or nausea, again, because the person believes they are taking some sort of medicine.

So in order to see if a therapy really works, there should be two groups of patients: half are given the treatment being tested, while half are given dummy pills, but neither group knows which treatment they are having. Then halfway through the trial the pills should be switched. It is what scientists call a 'double-blind crossover trial' and it can show clearly whether a therapy is different – or not – to dummy pills, whether it appears to alleviate symptoms, and also whether it causes more side effects.

The trouble is that this kind of trial is expensive (especially if you want to do it with the co operation of large numbers of patients), and it's something that manufacturers of alternative remedies simply can't afford to do on a large scale. So this means there just isn't the good evidence for alternative remedies that there is for conventional drugs, like HRT. Not only this, but there is an added problem that many alternative remedies contain different concentrations of ingredients, of differing purity. Until very recently there has been no legislation governing the purity of herbal remedies in the UK, or how they were manufactured, and this meant that some products did not necessarily contain what was stated on the label. So just because a trial on, for example, one product containing red clover leaf extract does not show any benefit, this does not mean that the same results can be applied to all red clover leaf products. But any scientific evidence is better than none at all, and probably the best way of judging whether a product works is to look at the results of several different trials all lumped together – what's known as a 'meta-analysis'.

Herbal remedies and food supplements – what's the difference?

All medicines now labelled as a 'herbal remedy' in the UK have to be registered with the Medicines and Healthcare products Regulatory Agency (MHRA). This confirms that they contain exactly what the packaging says they contain, that it has come from a guaranteed source and has been manufactured in a controlled way, just like regular medicines. The only difference from regular medicines is that there is no guarantee that they will work. However, they must come with an information leaflet that lists what is in the medicines, their potential side effects, and their interactions with other medicines.

Food supplements do not have any guarantee about the source or purity of their ingredients, and neither do they come with any information about side effects. They do, however, like all foods, have to be fit for human consumption.

Phytoestrogens

These are naturally occurring plant chemicals that have a weak oestrogen-like action. They are part of a group of chemicals known as isoflavones (a term you may see on labels), but of the thousand or so isoflavones found in plants, only four with oestrogen-like activity are found in the human diet – daidzein, genistein, formononetin and biochanin A. Rich sources of these include pulses, soy products and whole grains and seeds, including flaxseed, rye and millet. A wide range of supplements containing isoflavones are available, including those containing red clover, flaxseeds and those based on soya.

Phytoestrogens can bind to oestrogen receptors, but unlike the body's own oestrogen they do not have a direct stimulant action on all of them. Rather, they appear to somehow alter the action of some receptors, stimulating them in some areas of the body and blocking them elsewhere. It's what experts call a 'selective oestrogen receptor modulator', or SERM. Some conventional drugs act in this way, for example, the breast cancer treatment drug tamoxifen, which suppresses oestrogen receptors in the breast but stimulates them in bone (helping to prevent osteoporosis) and the uterus – promoting thickening of the womb lining and increasing the risk of endometrial cancer. The extent to which isoflavones exert oestrogenic actions on some tissues, and anti-oestrogenic actions on others, has led to a range of different health claims, including lowering the risk of heart disease, osteoporosis and breast cancer as well as relief from menopausal symptoms.

The bacteria that are found naturally in the large bowel play an important role in the metabolism of isoflavones, and the amount that is absorbed into the bloodstream. That means that the actual amount absorbed can vary widely from woman to woman, depending on the make-up of her natural gut organisms, and whether, for instance, she has recently taken antibiotics, which can reduce the number of bacteria present.

Some clinical trials have been done on supplements containing red clover, but the results have been variable. Some showed a moderate reduction in hot flushes, while in others it was no better than with a placebo pill. Reported side effects included rashes, muscle aches, headache, nausea and, more worryingly, vaginal spotting (which could have been due to thickening of the lining of the womb). Which brings me on to another issue; though a diet rich in isoflavones does appear to bring benefits, and is not harmful, the long-term safety of taking isoflavones in a concentrated supplement is not known, and some scientists argue that if there is enough active ingredient to actually make a difference, then it's akin to taking a form of HRT, and long-term effects need to be considered. In particular, it is simply not known whether taking isoflavone supplements long term could increase the risk of breast cancer, or cancer of the womb.

MY VERDICT: Try diet and lifestyle measures first. If these don't work and you are still having terrible hot flushes and want to avoid prescription drugs, an isoflavone-based remedy is worth a try. However, if you have had a hormone-dependent tumour, or a strong family history of these, such as breast cancer, please speak to your doctor first. If you do want to give isoflavones a try, make sure you buy a product with an MHRA herbal registration number.

Wild yam root

This is often advertised as a natural source of oestrogen and is promoted as a natural remedy for hot flushes and other menopausal symptoms. It contains diosgenin, a phytoestrogen, which in laboratories can be chemically converted into progesterone. Diosgenin was used to make the first oral contraceptive pills back in the 1960s. Unfortunately, studies have shown that taking wild yam supplements do not alter oestrogen or progesterone levels in the body, and there is little scientific evidence to support claims that it can help reduce hot flushes or other menopausal symptoms.

Creams containing wild yam are also available, but be warned, some of these have been found to contain synthetic hormones.

MY VERDICT: A waste of money.

Black cohosh

This herb, *Cimicifuga racemosa*, is a member of the buttercup family and has been used for centuries as a remedy for menstrual problems. The root, which is the part that is used, contains numerous different chemicals, including triterpene glycosides, flavonoids and aromatic acids. It does not have an oestrogenic mechanism of action, but rather appears to act on serotonin receptors. It has been claimed that black cohosh can help with a range of symptoms, including mood swings and depression as well as hot flushes. Evidence about both its effectiveness and safety is mixed – as with so many remedies, some studies show that it can be beneficial, while in others it is no better than a placebo. There have been no long-term safety studies, as most of the research that's been done has been in trials lasting less than six months. There have been some reports linking hepatitis and liver damage with the use of black cohosh-containing products, but it has not been proven that the herb is damaging, and some of the cases may have been due to using black cohosh that was grown in the wild and contaminated with harmful products from other plants.

Side effects from black cohosh can include stomach upsets and headaches.

MY VERDICT: Worth a try for hot flushes, but only for short-term relief. Don't use it for more than six months. With this herb it really is essential that you buy a registered product, so that its purity is guaranteed. Do not take it if you have a history of liver disorders, or if you are a heavy drinker. If you develop any signs of liver problems, such as yellowing of your skin, or dark urine, stop taking it straight away and see your GP.

Sage

This is a common herb, *Salvia officinalis*, that has been reported to ease menopausal sweating in particular. However, the few trials that have been done have failed to confirm it is any better than a placebo. Though it is considered safe for use as a food seasoning, some species of sage contain thujone, which can affect the nervous system. Taking extended or large doses of sage can cause restlessness, dizziness, vomiting, tremors and even seizures. It can also lead to wheezing and can cause skin rashes.

MY VERDICT: Much as I love it in food, this is not one to take for menopausal symptoms. There are less-risky alternatives.

Liquorice root

Liquorice root has traditionally been used for sore throats and chesty coughs, and more recently has been promoted as a remedy for hot flushes and sweats. It contains glycyrrhizin, and some short-term small trials have suggested it can help reduce hot flushes and sweats, but it can be more than a week before it takes effect. However, in large amounts it can cause high blood pressure, fluid retention and low blood levels of potassium. It can also reduce the levels of natural steroids, such as cortisol. The safety of taking supplements for more than six weeks has not been studied.

MY VERDICT: Small doses for the short term may be helpful. Definitely best avoided long term, though.

Grapeseed

Grapeseeds contain proanthocyanidin-a, which is an antioxidant. Grapeseed extract has traditionally been used to treat disorders of the heart and circulation, and more recently has been promoted as a remedy for menopausal symptoms. There have been very few studies on its efficacy in menopausal women, but it may have a slight beneficial effect on flushes, anxiety and depression. As with so many herbal remedies, trials have been short, but there have been no safety concerns if grapeseed is taken for up to eight weeks. Side effects reported include a dry itchy scalp, dizziness, headache and nausea.

MY VERDICT: Worth a try for troublesome flushes if other remedies have not helped.

Ginseng

Asian ginseng has been used to treat numerous different ailments for centuries, including boosting stamina and general wellbeing, improving the immune system and aiding recovery from illness, lowering blood glucose and also alleviating symptoms of the menopause.

The root of Asian ginseng contains chemicals known as ginsenosides, which are thought to be responsible for the claimed medicinal properties. Most of the medicinal claims for ginseng are based on research done in laboratories. Rather surprisingly, given its popularity, there is a paucity of large-scale clinical trials, though those that have been done do support claims that it may have a positive effect on immune function and lowering of blood glucose levels. Interestingly, the research that has been done suggests that ginseng may help with mood and sleep disturbances associated with the menopause, but it's not been shown to be helpful with hot flushes. Long-term use of ginseng has not been shown to be harmful but it can cause side effects including headaches and digestive disturbances. It can also cause allergic reactions. It should be avoided in those with diabetes who are taking other medicines to lower blood sugar.

MY VERDICT: If you need a boost of energy, or are suffering from mood swings, it is maybe worth a try, but don't expect it to reduce flushes or hot sweats.

Evening primrose oil

This is another remedy that has been promoted to help with 'women's problems' particularly premenstrual syndrome and also menopausal symptoms. The extract from its seeds contains gamma linoleic acid (GLA), an essential fatty acid. Sadly, there is little scientific research confirming that evening primrose oil makes a significant difference to menopausal conditions. There is no research on long-term safety, but it seems to be well tolerated by most people. Side effects can include nausea, diarrhoea and headaches. Evening primrose oil has active ingredients that can interact with the blood-thinning agent warfarin, and can induce seizures in those taking antipsychotic medication.

MY VERDICT: Don't waste your money.

Vitamin E

Taking supplements of vitamin E has been suggested as a possible treatment for flushes and sweats for the past 70 years. It's a fat-soluble vitamin that is found naturally in nuts, seeds and wheat germ and has several important functions, including protecting the membranes of cells in the body. Some women have reported that vitamin E supplements help relieve mild hot flushes, but scientific research has failed to prove that it's any better than a placebo. Taking a dose greater than 600mg a day may not be safe, as this may be associated with an increased risk of cardiovascular disease. But taking a dose less than this is unlikely to do any harm.

MY VERDICT: Worth a try for mild hot flushes, but if they are making your life a misery, you'll need something more effective. Read the label carefully and watch the dose you are taking.

Acupuncture

Chinese medicine has a long history of helping relieve the symptoms of the menopause, but they have different descriptions for different types of hot flushes. Before treating you, the specialist should take a careful history of your symptoms, do a thorough physical examination, looking especially at your tongue as well as your pulse. This is to determine whether you are having a 'hot' or 'cold' menopause and to tailor your treatment accordingly. Acupuncture aims to alter your Xi (your inner energy) by inserting needles in specific areas. Many practitioners combine acupuncture with a customised mix of herbal remedies, which are often based on the ingredients listed above.

Yet again, good scientific research is lacking to say whether it is any better than a placebo, but lots of women have said that acupuncture has helped them.

MY VERDICT: May be worth a try if you believe it could help you, but make sure you go to a reputable practitioner. Ask about the ingredients of any herbal remedies you have been given – don't take any concoction without knowing what's in it. Do not try to treat yourself with a mix of Chinese herbs you have bought yourself – if you want to go down the herbal remedy route, always buy registered products.

If you want information on St John's Wort and agnus castus, these are discussed in Chapter 4, as they are used primarily for regulating mood.

Sara, age 51

HER STORY: I haven't had a period for three months now, and I'm getting flushes and sweats. I try to keep fit and healthy, and go out running twice a week, which I think is helping. What else can I do? I really don't want to take pills – I want to manage this naturally. Would altering my diet help? It's already quite good, as I manage to get my five a day of fruit and veg, but I do like coffee from my espresso machine.

MY ADVICE: Cut down (slowly) on those caffeine-laden espressos – switch to decaf, and when making coffee at home, mix just a little normal coffee with decaf – many women say they don't really notice the difference. Avoid really hot, spicy food for a while, and keep an eye on your alcohol intake. These are the best dietary modifications that are likely to help reduce flushes and sweats.

It's also worth her trying to increase her intake of foods that contain phytoestrogens, which are weak oestrogen-like chemicals. These include pulses, linseeds and soya products, ideally having some of these every day. She could also substitute soya instead of meat in a lot of recipes, and with luck the rest of her family wouldn't notice! Simple things like changing to cotton underwear, wearing layers which are easy to peel off and having a really lightweight duvet with an extra blanket could help, too.

A couple of months later:

SARA: I've tried everything you said, but I'm still having loads of flushes and sweats, especially at night. I tried eating more seeds and soya, but the family started complaining about their food tasting different, and I don't think it made any difference to my flushes. I've also got new cotton undies and bedlinen, a light single duvet for me, but I think I need something more powerful. Are there any pills available other than HRT? I'd prefer to keep that as a last resort as my mother had breast cancer.

MY ADVICE: I suggested she try a low dose of an antidepressant, even though she hadn't mentioned depression, or even mood swings, these drugs can act on the centre in the brain that controls temperature and can help hot flushes and sweats. These drugs don't work for all women, but they are worth a try for those who want to avoid HRT. Starting with 10mg citalopram a day for a couple of weeks may be enough, but if she still got flushes and sweats, I suggested we could increase it to 20mg. The drugs should start working within a few days, but I warned her that during this time she may get side effects,

THE DREADED FLUSHES AND SWEATS

such as slight nausea, and a dry mouth. She might also feel a
bit more anxious, but she should try to stick with it, and then
in a couple of weeks hopefully she would be feeling a lot more
comfortable.

HER DECISION: She decided to give low-dose antidepressants a
try. I had a telephone consultation six weeks later and she said
that they had definitely taken the edge off both the flushes and
sweats, and that she was sleeping a lot better. So she decided
to stick with them for the next few months.

Gill, age 50

HER STORY: I'm sure I'm in the change. My periods are completely
erratic – I never know when I'm going to have one. I can cope
with that – just – but the flushes and sweats are getting me
down. I've thought about HRT, but my friends who have tried
it have said that it's made them put on weight, and at my size,
that's the last thing I want! Is there anything else I can do?

MY ADVICE: Losing weight will help hot flushes and sweats, and
to do that successfully she would need to increase the amount
of exercise she did – which would help as well. Switching
polyester clothes for cotton ones, eating more soya products,
cutting down on coffee and especially alcohol – since it's full
of empty calories would also help. I suggested she try just that
approach for a few weeks, but if she wanted to try something
else there were other medicines, like antidepressants, or
herbal remedies.

HER DECISION: She really didn't like the idea of going on
antidepressants, and she thought that knowing that losing

weight would help her flushes and sweats would give her an extra incentive to go on a diet, and stick to it.

FOLLOW-UP: She came back to see me again six weeks later. She was exercising more and had lost half a stone, she had boosted her soya intake, too, and her flushes weren't quite so bad.

But she was still having a lot of them and wanted something else to help. However, she didn't like the idea of either HRT or antidepressants and wanted more information about herbal remedies.

She decided to try black cohosh and made sure she bought a reputable registered brand. It did help with her flushes, which gradually reduced in severity, and she was able to stop taking it after six months. She still had occasional sweats afterwards, but she felt able to cope with them without any further medication.

SUMMARY

Flushes and sweats are often the most troubling symptoms of the menopause. Not all women get them, but in some they are so severe that they make life a misery.

The exact cause isn't known, but it's thought that the fall in oestrogen levels at the menopause affects the centre in the brain that controls body temperature. This effect is in part controlled by the chemical messengers serotonin and noradrenaline.

Flushes and sweats usually start as oestrogen levels begin to fall in the perimenopause, though they may not start until periods actually stop. They are usually at their worst for the first six months to a year, but there is no way of predicting how long they are going to continue. Some women only get them for a couple of months, in others they go on for years.

- Lifestyle changes can help, particularly wearing layers of clothing made of natural fabrics which don't hold sweat. Bedlinen made of 100 per cent cotton can make nights more comfortable than poly-cotton mixed fabrics.

- Cutting down on alcohol, coffee and spicy foods can also help, and getting into the habit of taking regular exercise can make a difference, too.

- Drugs that boost serotonin and noradrenaline levels, which are traditionally used to treat depression and anxiety, have been found to help reduce flushes and sweats.

- Foods rich in isoflavones, which have a weak oestrogen-like action, can sometimes reduce flushes and sweats a little.

- A wide range of alternative remedies are available, though they may have very little effect. The best ones are those containing phytoestrogens, and black cohosh can be helpful, too, but should not be taken for more than six months. It is important to only use registered herbal products and not take any labelled as food supplements, which have no guarantee of the purity of their ingredients.

- And then there is HRT. This is such a big topic it has its own chapter – and that's coming next.

3

HORMONE REPLACEMENT THERAPY

Nearly all the women who come to see me at the time of the menopause want information about HRT. A few are determined to avoid it, but the majority want to know what it will do for them – the benefits and also, very importantly, the risks.

So what I'll try to do in this chapter is guide you through the maze that is HRT – giving you the information you will need to help you make an informed choice about whether or not you want to give it a try.

In the first part of this chapter you'll find basic information about HRT, followed by more details about the various different types of HRT and the differences between them. Then, as with other chapters, there are some sections with extra scientific information and research data, if you want to know more about this. I've also included some case histories, starting on page 88, to give you practical advice on how HRT can work for individual women. If you like, you can go straight to this section and then check back for further information.

SO, WHAT IS HRT?

As its name suggests, Hormone Replacement Therapy – HRT – replaces the hormones that are no longer being produced by the ovaries.

The main ingredient is oestrogen, the hormone that the body misses so much, and the aim of HRT is to restore oestrogen levels, allowing the body to function as it did before the menopause.

Using oestrogen alone can cause thickening of the endometrium (the lining of the womb) which in the long term can cause erratic bleeding and the development of abnormal cells, increasing the risk of cancer of the womb. This can be counteracted by adding in a progestogen, a synthetic form of the natural form of the hormone progesterone which ensures the womb lining remains safe. For more detail about this, see page 76.

Hattie, age 50

'I was all set to try to manage my menopause myself, and hoped I could cope by altering my diet and taking more exercise. But I kept an open mind about HRT, which was just as well. My body thermostat seemed to go completely out of control – one moment I was hot, the next I was cold, I couldn't sleep, and I just didn't feel like having sex any more. It would be wrong to say life wasn't worth living any more, but I was really miserable. HRT was a saviour for me. I decided to go for the straightforward 'pill' option, and though to begin with it meant having periods again, they weren't that heavy, and I could alter the time they occurred. I did feel a bit bloated to begin with, and did find controlling my weight a bit more tricky, but I had far more energy than before, and fancied my husband again. I reckon my complexion looks a bit better as well. I know there are some health risks with HRT, but for me, they were worth it. It gave me back a normal life.'

What are the advantages?

There are two very important benefits of HRT. The first is that it is an extremely effective way of controlling hot flushes and sweats and for this reason alone, most women taking HRT say that this benefit makes a significant difference to their quality of life and wellbeing.

The second important benefit of HRT is that it can reduce the risk of developing osteoporosis. The effect mainly occurs while HRT is being taken, but although bone density falls after stopping HRT, some studies have shown that women who take HRT for a few years around the time of the menopause may have gained a small long-term protective effect on their bones.

Anything else?

There have been some scientific studies that suggest HRT improves skin and hair thickness and helps maintain the strength and moisture of the tissues in the genital area. Through an action on oestrogen receptors in the brain, it can also help with mood swings, depression and anxiety that can occur around the time of the change. Other women report it improves muscle aches and pains. Many women say it improves their vitality and libido, and just makes them feel normal again.

In other words, it puts their body back to where it was before the menopause.

And to add to the good news, there is also good evidence that it can slightly help reduce the risk of cancer of the colon and rectum.

How long does it take to work?

Flushes and sweats start to reduce within days of starting HRT, and there is usually a significant reduction in hot flushes and sweats within four weeks, but maximum benefit may take three months. Compared with placebo pills, HRT reduces flushes by 87 per cent after four months of use.

What about Alzheimer's? And heart disease?

There have been other beneficial claims about HRT, the most controversial of which is that it may help protect against Alzheimer's disease and preserve memory. However, the research doesn't fully back this up, and as yet there is no good evidence that HRT can delay the onset or slow down the progress of Alzheimer's.

So what about the disadvantages?

There are two main reasons why HRT has fallen out of favour; there is no doubt that it can increase the risk of both breast cancer and blood clots, and to add to the bad news, more recently evidence has emerged that it can also increase the risk of ovarian cancer.

But is it really that dangerous?

No. Far too many women have been put off – or even refused – HRT because the risks have been exaggerated. The increased risk of getting breast cancer is really very small, and there is more information about this on page 64.

The increased risk of blood clots is also very small – and miniscule with HRT that you apply via your skin. See page 66 for more information on this.

In other words, HRT is NOT necessarily the baddy it is so often made out to be.

Is it true that HRT can make you put on weight? What about other side effects?

Both the oestrogen and progestogen components of HRT can cause side effects.

Possible side effects of oestrogen include:

- fluid retention, leading to bloating

- breast tenderness and swelling

- nausea

- leg cramps

- headaches

- indigestion.

And possible side effects of progestogen include:

- fluid retention

- breast tenderness

- headaches

- mood swings and depression

- greasy skin and acne.

As with all drug side effects, some women taking HRT don't get any of them, while others aren't so lucky. All are dose dependent – the higher the dose, the worse the side effects are likely to be. Side effects can also vary according to the type of oestrogen and progestogen used, and also the route of administration. If one type of HRT does not suit you, it's worth trying a different one, either in the form of a different hormone, or a different formulation. (There is more information about this on pages 80 and also in the section on case histories, starting on page 88.)

MORE SCIENTIFIC INFORMATION

The oestrogens in HRT

The oestrogens used in HRT are usually referred to as 'natural' because they resemble the substances produced by the body. They include oestradiol, oestrone and oestriol, which are usually made from either soya beans or yam extracts. 'Conjugated equine oestrogens', which are found in some types of HRT, are made from the urine of pregnant horses, which is high in oestrone sulphate.

Breast cancer

There is no doubt that taking HRT increases, very slightly, the risk of breast cancer. Most research studies suggest that oestrogen is the main culprit, but a recent study has suggested that progesterone may be more important. What the studies do agree on is that the increased risk of breast cancer rises the longer you take HRT, and also with the size of the dose – the higher the dose of oestrogen, the greater the risk. And taking both progesterone and oestrogen raises the risk more than taking oestrogen alone. But that said, the absolute risks of HRT are actually very small. It works out at about one extra case of breast cancer per 1,000 women each year. That is about the same as drinking two to three units of alcohol a day – which many women do without thinking of breast cancer. It's also similar to the risk of being overweight, or not having had children, starting your periods early or having a late menopause (all of which increase the risk of breast cancer).

Here's a table which shows the risks:

Using HRT for 5 and 10 years between the ages of 50 and 54

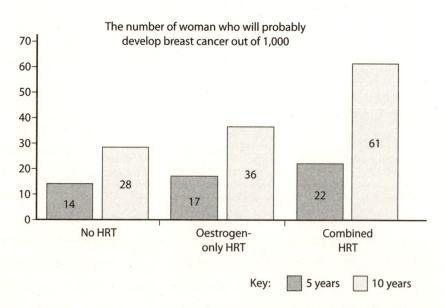

The number of woman who will probably develop breast cancer out of 1,000

No HRT: 14 (5 years), 28 (10 years)
Oestrogen-only HRT: 17 (5 years), 36 (10 years)
Combined HRT: 22 (5 years), 61 (10 years)

Key: 5 years / 10 years

figures taken from Breast Cancer Now Generations Study

Having seen this, it might be tempting to take oestrogen without any added progesterone. However, oestrogen alone causes an increase in the risk of cancer of the lining of the womb, so it is never done. The best way of protecting the womb lining, and giving minimal progesterone to the breasts, is almost certainly to have a Mirena coil fitted, but as yet there is no long-term data on the increased risk of breast cancer with this method.

HRT, osteoporosis and bowel cancer

The effect of HRT on bones is dose-dependent – the higher the dose, the better the effect on bones. Some low-dose formulations only have a slight impact on bones, and do not entirely prevent osteoporosis. In the large Women's Health Initiative (WHI) trial on HRT (discussed in more detail on page 66), women taking combined oestrogen and progesterone HRT in a standard dose had one-third fewer hip and vertebral (backbone) fractures per year compared to those taking placebo tablets. In absolute terms, this translates to 10 fractures per 10,000 women who took HRT, compared to 15 fractures per 10,000 women in those taking placebo.

In the same trial, HRT reduced the risk of bowel cancer by one-third, translating to 10 cases of colorectal cancer per 10,000 women who took HRT compared to 16 per 10,000 in those who took placebo.

Alzheimer's

A review by the Cochrane group (a large independent advisory panel) done in 2008 came to the conclusion that there was no good evidence that HRT prevented cognitive decline either in the short or longer term (up to five years). The biggest risk factor for Alzheimer's disease is carriage of certain genes, especially one known as the APOE e4 variant. People with one copy of this gene (estimated to be about one in four) have a four times increased risk of Alzheimer's, and those with two copies (one from each parent), which is around one in 50 people, have a ten-fold increase. The Cochrane review did not look at the effect of HRT on APOE e4 carriers, and some small studies done more recently have suggested that HRT may help slow down cellular ageing in carriers.

Heart disease

Some data does exist that suggests that HRT may reduce the risk of heart disease in the first few years after the menopause, but to put this in context, the risk of heart disease in women in their late forties and early fifties is very low. Larger trials on older women, in their late fifties, taking HRT compared to those not taking HRT have suggested that HRT might slightly increase the risk of heart disease.

So, overall, it is now thought that HRT is not going to make a significant difference to heart disease risk, and other factors – such as smoking, weight, blood pressure, exercise and cholesterol level – are way more important.

Blood clots

Taking HRT by mouth increases the risk of blood clots occurring in veins, both in deep veins (a deep vein thrombosis, or DVT), in the lungs (a pulmonary embolus) and also in the veins of the brain, which can lead to stroke. The risk appears to be greatest in the first year of use, and also increases with the age of the woman and with other risk factors for clots, such as obesity, smoking, a family history of clots and being immobile. As with breast cancer, the addition of a progestogen increases the risk, especially if the progestogen medroxyprogesterone acetate is used.

The big research trials

Many large studies have been carried out in the last twenty years, but the two most important ones are the Women's Health Initiative

(WHI) study which took place in the USA, and the Million Women Study which was conducted in the UK.

The Women's Health Initiative was started in the USA in 1993. It was designed to look at major health problems affecting post-menopausal women, including breast cancer, strokes and heart disease, and how these were affected by taking HRT. It was a complex trial with several different components, one of which involved some women being deliberately given HRT, to compare with those who were not. More than 160,000 women, aged between 50 and 79, took part in the study over 15 years.

The Million Women Study was a British study of women's health using data from more than a million women aged 50 and over, led by Dame Valerie Beral and her team of researchers at the University of Oxford. It has received funding from Cancer Research UK, the NHS and also the Medical Research Council. One important part of the study was to look at the effects of HRT.

Both trials confirmed that women taking HRT had a greater risk of breast cancer compared to those who did not, and that taking both oestrogen and progestogen (combined HRT) carried a greater risk than oestrogen alone. The results were so clear-cut that one part of the WHI trial had to be stopped four years early, as it was felt that women given HRT were being put at an unacceptable risk compared to those who were not. The Million Women Study suggested that the risks for breast cancer were similar for all types of oestrogen and progestogen, including oral, transdermal and implanted HRT, though the use of the Mirena coil for the progestogen component was not studied.

Though HRT (both oestrogen only and combined) increases the risk of stroke due to venous clots, unlike breast cancer the risk does not appear to continue rising in those over 60, except with one type of HRT known as Tibolone, which appears to have double the risk of stroke compared to women not taking HRT.

Both trials led to sensational headlines and many inaccurate reports, which had a real scaremongering effect on women. As with all trials, there were drawbacks – many of the women in them were in their sixties and seventies, and were given higher doses of HRT than would be used today. Many of the reports expressed the risk in terms of 'percentage increase', but these single numbers can be very misleading, as any calculation of increased risk should take into account each individual's pre-existing risk of contracting breast cancer, as shown by their background.

In the summer of 2016, data from another large study was published. Carried out in the UK by the Institute of Cancer Research and the National Cancer Registration and Analysis Service, this studied just under 40,000 women over six years, and the results suggested that the previous studies had underestimated the increased risk of breast cancer caused by taking HRT, and that taking combined HRT for just over five years doubled the risk of breast cancer, and after 15 years the risk rose to over three times compared to those who never took HRT. Interestingly, though, this study suggested there was no increased risk with oestrogen – only HRT.

However, the overall number of women in the study who developed breast cancer was small – 52 – and of these, only seven had been taking HRT for 15 years. So many experts say they think the results of the older trials give more accurate information.

So that's the background to HRT.

In the next section I'll explain about the different types of HRT available.

I'll start with the questions that I'm often asked, and then give some more detailed background information.

What types of HRT are available?

There are two main routes of administering HRT: by mouth, as tablets, and via the skin, in the form of patches or gels. Oestrogen is also available as implants, placed under the skin, which release hormones gradually over a period of six months. However, these are far less popular now than they used to be.

If you need progesterone as well, this can be given either as tablets or patches or directly to the womb via a Mirena coil.

What is the difference between them?

First, there are different types of oestrogen, in differing doses, then there is the progesterone component to consider.

Is one type better than another?

The different ways in which oestrogen is given can have differing effects on the body, for instance, on blood-clotting factors – oestrogen given via the skin does not increase the risk of a stroke, and this is very important for some women. Many women also say they get less side effects with patches or gel, and it's easy to adjust the dose with gel. However, as always, the most important thing is that you have a type of HRT that suits you – and that may well be different from the type that suits your best friend!

The Mirena coil? Isn't that a contraceptive – which I don't need at my age?

The Mirena is small T-shaped device which looks very similar to a copper intra-uterine contraceptive device. It has a core of the progestogen around the long arm of the T, which is slowly released into the womb lining over a period of five years. With a Mirena in place, any type of oestrogen can be used to help control menopausal symptoms. This means that the dose and route of oestrogen can be tailored to a woman's individual needs. An added advantage of the Mirena is that the amount of progesterone absorbed into the general circulation is very small, which minimises progestogenic side effects. In theory, using a Mirena may also reduce the added risk of breast cancer that progesterone brings to an HRT regime, but there is no confirmatory data on this.

Angie, age 51

'I was a bit surprised when my GP suggested I should have a
Mirena coil as part of my HRT. After all, one of the few good
things I was looking forward to with the menopause was not
having to bother about contraception any more! But then, I
didn't fancy having periods back, and that was what other forms
of HRT would have entailed. So I opted for gel for the oestrogen
that my body seemed to be crying out for, and a Mirena to
protect my womb lining. My GP was really honest with me about
the fitting – she warned me that it would be uncomfortable, but
actually, it wasn't that bad. I've had three kids, so maybe that
has altered my pain threshold when it comes to my "gynae area"
but it was only a bit more uncomfortable than having a smear
taken. I had some cramps afterwards for a couple of days but
all I needed was a couple of ibuprofen. I was still having erratic
periods when I started HRT, and I did have some bleeding for a
few weeks after it was put in, but it wasn't heavy. And then my
periods stopped completely, and I didn't get any side effects
from either the device, or the hormones it was releasing. My
husband said he couldn't feel the threads during sex, which I
was concerned about beforehand, so I had all the advantages of
HRT, but no progesterone–related disadvantages, like periods or
greasy skin. It's been a good method for me.'

Are there lots of different types of tablets? What's the difference between them?

Yes, tablets come in a range of doses, containing between 1 and 2mg
of estradiol valerate or plain estradiol, or between 0.3mg and 1.25mg
of conjugated oestrogens. There is also one preparation that contains
a mix of three different oestrogens: estriol, estradiol and estrone.

For women who need progesterone as well, tablets may contain just oestrogen, or both oestrogen and a progestogen. Some come in 'cyclical packs' where just oestrogen is taken for two weeks, then a pill containing both oestrogen and a progestogen (which are a different colour) are taken for a further two weeks.

As well as the progestogens available as part of a ready-made therapy, progestogen tablets can also be prescribed completely separately, to be taken cyclically for two weeks each month, with an oestrogen-only preparation being used all the time.

What about patches and gels?

Patches are applied to the skin and changed either once or twice a week, while gels are applied either as a premeasured sachet-full or 'blob'. The hormones are absorbed directly through the skin into the bloodstream and, unlike tablets, there does not seem to be a significant increased risk of developing blood clots. There are also reports that gastrointestinal side effects, such as nausea, are less common with patches, and that mood swings may be less, as the patches give a constant level of hormone in the bloodstream.

But don't patches come off? What about allergic reactions?

Yes, the adhesive in the patches can cause irritation of the skin and, like any plaster, they can leave a sticky mark after they are removed. They generally stick on very well and don't come off when you wash, or go swimming, but if you put them under the edge of clothing, for example a belt, they may roll at the corners. They release a constant amount of hormone throughout the time they are applied, so if a patch comes off you just apply another one.

Are patches better if you have had a medical condition or are taking other medicines?

Transdermal preparations are often more suitable for women who have a history of liver disease or gallstones, those with diabetes, and those taking medicines that can affect liver enzymes (such as some pain relief and anti-convulsant drugs). They can also be a better option for women who suffer migraines that are triggered by the sudden surge in hormone levels that can occur with tablets.

Katie, age 51

'I'm hopeless at remembering to take tablets, so I liked the idea of patches that I would only need to change once a week. To begin with I put them on my buttock, but the edges tended to roll when I took my jeans on and off. My lower tummy seemed a better place. I didn't have any problems with skin irritation, though sometimes my skin did feel a bit sticky when I took one off. They worked really well at relieving my flushes, and also my attacks of anxiety, and the only side effect I had was a bit of weight gain. I need to work on that, but otherwise they suited me really well.'

When can you start HRT? Do you have to wait until your periods have stopped?

The time most women start HRT is when they are getting bad flushes or sweats, and this can be before, or after, your periods have stopped. (There is more information about starting HRT on page 75.)

What about the progesterone bit?

All progesterones used in HRT are synthetic – that is, made in a laboratory, and known as progestogens. There are two main types of progestogen used in HRT: those that closely resemble natural progesterone and those derived from testosterone – norethisterone, norgestrel and levonorgestrel.

Do you need to take progesterone all the time?

It depends on the type of HRT regime you are taking. The progesterone component can be given either cyclically or all the time. In perimenopausal women, and those within a year of their last period who still may have some natural ovarian activity, it is given for two weeks each month, after which there is a withdrawal bleed. This means that women on this type of regime have a monthly 'period'. However, the combination of hormones used can be adjusted to try to avoid this being too heavy.

For other women, whose last period was more than a year ago, a 'continuous combined' preparation is usually used, which contains a constant amount of both hormones, which are taken all the time. Though this can cause some erratic bleeding to begin with, after a few months there should be no bleeding at all – in other words, no periods.

I've had a hysterectomy, do I still need to take progesterone?

No. Women who have had a hysterectomy only need oestrogen, as the only reason for adding in the progesterone component is to protect the womb lining.

What about side effects?

Side effects apart from bleeding, such as bloating, nausea and breast tenderness, always tend to be worse in the first few weeks of treatment. As the body adapts and gets used to the raised levels of oestrogen, they usually settle down. But if they persist, go back to see your doctor and discuss changing to either a different type of oestrogen, progestogen, or both. Some women develop PMS-type symptoms on some types of cyclical regime, especially if the preparation contains norethisterone, norgestrel or levonorgestrel, which are chemically similar to testosterone. It can help to switch to one with less testosterone-like activity, such as medroxyprogesterone acetate or dydrogesterone.

Are there any women who really should not have HRT?

Some other health issues can mean it is simply too dangerous for particular women to have HRT, as any benefits of HRT are outweighed by the risks.

These include:

- Most women who have had breast cancer

- Most women who have had endometrial cancer, or other cancers that are oestrogen-dependent

- Most women with a history of a venous blood clot

- Uncontrolled high blood pressure – but you can take HRT if your blood pressure is well controlled with medication

- Active liver disease, with abnormal liver function tests

- A recent heart attack, or ongoing symptoms of a reduced blood supply to the heart.

You'll see that I've put 'most women' in a few places. Occasionally women with what used to be regarded as an absolute contra-indication to HRT, and who are desperate to have it, are given it in certain circumstances. But this is a decision that is only ever taken by an expert, and the women concerned may have to sign a disclaimer saying they are prepared to take responsibility for the risks involved.

So what's your view of HRT? Do you prescribe it?

There is no doubt that HRT is the best way to relieve unpleasant menopausal symptoms. I think it's had an unfair negative press and it's not the 'baddy' that it is often made out to be, and if flushes, sweats and sleepless nights are making your life a misery it's well worth considering. And yes, I prescribe lots of HRT.

However, it's important to weigh up any other factors that may also be putting you at increased risk of breast cancer or strokes – for example, do you have a family history of these conditions? Are you overweight? Do you drink more than 14 units of alcohol a week? (be honest...). All these factors can add up and make taking HRT that little bit more of a risk to your health. In the end, though, it's up to each individual woman to make up her own mind, though of course it helps to have a really good doctor who can give you balanced expert advice.

HRT can also be a really good option for women in their fifties who are at increased risk of osteoporosis. There is more information about this in Chapter 6.

STARTING HRT – CHOOSING YOUR PREPARATION

Philippa, age 55

'I really didn't know very much about HRT before I went to see my doctor – all I knew was that I needed something to sort out my horrendous flushes and sweats, and that would help me to be able to sleep and feel normal again. I had no idea I needed two hormones – I thought I only needed replacement oestrogen – so the whole business of having progesterone and having periods again came as a surprise. My doctor went through all the different types of HRT, but I just couldn't take it all in, there and then, or decide what I wanted. So she printed out some information for me to read at home. Even then, I still needed to go through it all twice to get my head around all the facts. I went back again a couple of weeks later, and then it was much easier to discuss the pro and cons of each method. I was lucky that I had an understanding doctor – I reckon some GPs would just give you pills and not explain all the other options that are available. So I

> really would advise any woman who is thinking of HRT to do some homework about it first. There's no way a doctor can give you all the information you need to know to make an informed choice in a standard 10-minute appointment.'

Before you can start HRT your blood pressure will need to be checked; if it is raised it will need to be brought under control before the drugs can be prescribed to you. As side effects are generally dose-related, it's best to start with a low-dose formulation, then give it a couple of months and see how you feel. Whether you have tablets, patches or gel is largely a matter of personal preference. Tablets are often regarded as the easiest to take, but many women say they get fewer side effects with gel or patches. These are safer in terms of not increasing your risk of a DVT, and gel also has the advantage of finer tuning of the dose – it's possible to put on half a blob, if that's all you need to control flushes and sweats. If you find that a low-dose preparation does not control your symptoms, then it's reasonable to increase to a higher dose.

ADDING IN THE PROGESTERONE

Unless you have had your womb removed, you will need to take additional progesterone, to prevent the oestrogen leading to a thickened lining. This can be given in one of three ways:

– If you are within a year of your last period you will need to take cyclical progesterone for two weeks each month. When you stop the progesterone you will have a withdrawal bleed, like a period. Depending on the type and dose of both oestrogen and progestogen, this may be light or heavy, and some women also get period pains. As with all hormone preparations, you need to give your body time to adjust to the new hormones it's being given, so it's best to try to stick with a regime for three months and see how it works. If you get a heavy or painful period, try not to give up on the regime straight away, but wait to see if things settle down and the next one is better. If things don't improve, try something different. Many women need to try three (and sometimes a lot more) different regimes before they find a hormone mix that suits them. Some women develop PMS-type symptoms on certain cyclical regimes, especially if the preparation contains norethisterone, norgestrel or levonorgestrel, which are chemically similar to testosterone. It can help to switch to one with less testosterone-like activity, such as medroxyprogesterone acetate or dydrogesterone.

– If it is more than a year since your last period, you can have a 'continuous combined' regime, which involves taking oestrogen and a low dose of progestogen all the time. This holds the lining of the womb in check and keeps it thin, which means you should not have any periods at all – which of course nearly all women prefer! The reason continuous combined regimes are not used in the perimenopause or immediately after periods have stopped is because there can be some residual ovarian activity, and this can lead occasionally to erratic heavy bleeding. So continuous combined regimes are only suitable for women who are assumed to have completely non-functioning ovaries. Both hormones are usually combined into a single pill or patch. However, as with cyclical regimes, it can take several months for the womb to get used to the hormones, and some bleeding is quite common in the first few months. It does not occur in a cyclical fashion, and can be very erratic, but it should not be heavy, and there certainly should not be clots. As with cyclical regimes, give each hormone mix at least three months for things to settle down.

– The other option is to have a Mirena coil device fitted to provide the progestogen component. The device slowly releases progesterone right where it's needed, into the womb lining. This means it's perfectly safe to just have oestrogen – the progestogen from the coil will protect the womb lining.

Timing the withdrawal bleed

Rachel, age 54

'I hadn't realised that taking HRT would mean having periods again, and I dreaded having to cope with them when I was on holiday. Thankfully my GP told me how I could alter the timing of when I bled, but I couldn't have done it straight away – I needed to experience how my body reacted to the hormones, and when the bleeding actually occurred in relation to the two different tablets I was taking. But once I'd got my head around that, it was quite easy to have my period when it suited me, though it did mean sometimes taking half a packet of pills, then throwing the rest away – which seemed a bit wasteful.'

If you are on a cyclical regime, it is possible to alter the timing of the 'withdrawal bleed' by simply delaying taking the progestogen-containing pills (or patches). This can be useful if you want to avoid having a period while you are on holiday. However, it should not be done for more than a couple of weeks, or repeatedly, as the overall higher dose of oestrogen compared to progestogen can lead to a build-up in the womb lining, which can not only lead to heavy bleeding, but theoretically might slightly increase the risk of endometrial cancer.

It is possible to alter a cyclical regime so you only have periods once every three months. This involves taking just oestrogen for 10 weeks, then a high dose of progesterone along with the oestrogen for the next two weeks. The withdrawal bleed from this type of regime tends to be quite heavy, so in my experience it is not usually a popular option. If you are only taking a very small dose of oestrogen, say a blob of gel every other day, it may be safe to only take progesterone once every two months, but this is something you need to discuss with your doctor.

CONTINUING HRT ... AND STOPPING

Wendy, age 58

'When I first started HRT, I just wanted to feel normal again. The question of how and when I was going to stop it was something for the future. HRT suited me really well, but as the years went by, and I saw my doctor for my annual check-ups, I realised, sadly, that I couldn't stay on it forever. My doctor was sympathetic, but clearly my sixtieth birthday was a cut-off point for her – after that the risks were just too great for her to carry on giving me prescriptions. I found the concept of having a stroke difficult to take on board, after all, that happened to older people, and I didn't feel remotely old. But I had to accept her advice.

'If I'm honest, coming off HRT was awful. I followed my doctor's advice and did it slowly, gradually reducing the dose, but I still got a few hot flushes and sweats, and my libido disappeared. I suspect there may have been a bit of a psychological element to this as I was no longer taking my "youth pills" and I was worried I was suddenly going to turn into some haggard old witch. But now, two years on, actually I'm OK. My skin is drier, and my sex drive isn't the same, but I pile on the moisturiser and I reckon I look fine for my age. And I have my health, and can still play tennis, and look after my new grandchild, and that's got to be better than having a stroke, or heart attack.'

Once you are settled on an HRT regime – and this can take time and a lot of trial and error – you should see your doctor once a year. This is to check your blood pressure, and also to check whether it is still the best regime for you, as new treatments are constantly being introduced. The other reason for the annual check is to discuss the pros and cons of continuing HRT. How long you continue with HRT is, like the decision to start it, very much a matter of personal choice. The standard recommendation is to take it for a short time, to get you through the worst of the symptoms that occur while the ovaries stop functioning, and in the immediate aftermath. Exactly how long this is varies from woman to woman, and in particular depends on when they started taking it. Those who start HRT before their periods stop may need to continue it for longer than a woman who starts it some months after her last period. In general, after two years, natural ovarian production of hormones will have stopped, and in theory this means that menopausal symptoms should have stopped. However, suddenly stopping HRT inevitably leads to a sudden drop in oestrogen levels, and this can trigger flushes and sweats all over again. For this reason, HRT should be tailed off slowly, so the body adapts to the falling oestrogen levels. Those on a high dose of oestrogen (a tablet containing 2mg oestradiol or a 75 or 100mcg patch) should switch to a lower-dose formulation. Just this switch alone can trigger some flushes and sweats, so you need to persevere until your body adapts – normally about three months. Once on a low dose, it can be helpful to take the oestrogen on alternate days, again for two or three months, before finally stopping. If withdrawal flushes or sweats are severe, taking an SSRI antidepressant, or clonidine tablets can be helpful.

What if you are happy on HRT and don't want to stop?

There are no set rules about how long you can take HRT and when you should stop. I have had a lot of patients who say they feel so well on HRT that they really don't want to come off it. The risks and benefits vary for each individual woman. Some are understandably worried about a recurrence of awful flushes and sweats, while others attribute their energy, or thick hair or good complexion to HRT. However, the increased risk of breast cancer and strokes (for oral treatments) mean that most doctors, especially GPs, are reluctant to continue prescribing it to women after the age of 60. That said, even in this age group in some, the benefits can still outweigh the risks, but any women continuing with it after 60 should transfer to a transdermal route (either patches or gel) as this has a lower risk of stroke compared to tablets. And beyond 70, the increased risk of breast cancer and stroke mean that the risks definitely outweigh any benefits, which means that HRT should be stopped.

What about contraception?

HRT is not a contraceptive – unlike the Pill, the levels of hormones are too low to override the natural activity of the ovaries. Though the risk of a pregnancy is low by the time a woman reaches the menopause, ovulation can still occur – often randomly and unpredictably. Experts say that a woman can be considered to be potentially fertile until a year after her last natural period, and that you need to carry on using contraception during this time. Of course, if you start taking HRT before your periods stop, working out when this is can be nigh on impossible, but it can help to have a 'pre-treatment' FSH level test to give an indication of your ovarian function. If you were having erratic periods and raging flushes and sweats, I think it's reasonable to assume that a year on you are highly unlikely to be producing any eggs, and it's reasonable to stop using contraception.

One very good option for contraception in perimenopausal women taking HRT is the Mirena device, which also provides the progesterone component, so all you need to have, HRT-wise, is straight oestrogen.

Women who have no other underlying health problems (for example, high blood pressure, diabetes, obesity) can usually take the contraceptive pill up until the age of 50. The combined pill, which contains oestrogen, overrides the natural ovarian function and stops ovulation. This also sometimes happens with the most commonly prescribed progesterone-only pill, which contains desogestrel. From your late forties onwards it can be impossible to know whether your ovaries will start working again when you stop the Pill, and the only way to find out is to 'try it and see'. If you suddenly have flushes and sweats, you have your answer! But it's still best to use a barrier method of contraception (condoms or a diaphragm) until you have had no periods for a year.

PREMATURE MENOPAUSE

Annie, age 45

'It was a real shock when I found out, at the age of 35, that my ovaries had stopped working and that I was menopausal. My GP was pretty insistent that I should take HRT, which I found a bit tricky, as everything I'd read about it suggested it should come with a major health warning. But she explained that in my case it would be replacing the hormones that my own body should still be producing, and that it was vital for keeping my bones strong – and also for maintaining a normal sex life. Quite frankly, when you hear that your ovaries aren't working in your thirties, libido isn't exactly the item top of the agenda, but I realise now she had a point. My second daughter was only three when my ovaries packed up, and thinking back, I don't think I'd have coped if I hadn't had the pills. I started sleeping normally again, and stopped losing my rag over silly little things. Weirdly, though, I think it was still having periods again that helped most of all – still having a "monthly" made me somehow feel normal again.'

Women who have an early menopause, where periods stop before the age of 45, are at increased risk of osteoporosis and also are likely to get symptoms of a dry vagina at a relatively young age. So, generally, for these women the benefits of HRT outweigh the risks, at least up until the age of 50. It is also a good idea for younger women to take a full 'bone-protective' dose of oestrogen (either a 2mg tablet, or 75 or 100mcg patch), to help prevent osteoporosis.

SOME BACKGROUND SCIENCE – OESTROGEN AND BLOOD CLOTS

The active ingredients in tablets reach the bloodstream after first being absorbed from the gut, then passing through the liver. It is thought that this 'first pass effect' through the liver influences the levels of blood-clotting factors and accounts for the increased risk of blood clots seen in the WHI and Million Women trials.

Some other options

Tibolone is a slightly different type of oral HRT. It combines both oestrogenic and progestogenic properties with a weak androgenic (testosterone-like) activity. Trials have shown that it can help relieve flushes and sweats, but is less effective than conventional HRT. It can help maintain bone density and it may help improve libido after the menopause. It does however carry an increased risk of stroke, and this means that in women over 60 (who have an increased risk of stroke simply because of their age) the risks outweigh any benefits.

Duavive is a new combination HRT tablet. The oestrogen in Duavive is a combination of three different types, aiming to replicate the oestrogens previously produced by the ovaries. The big difference is in the second hormone. Instead of a progesterone, Duavive contains bazedoxifene, a type of drug known as a selective oestrogen receptor modulator, or SERM. This blocks the action of oestrogen on the womb, preventing a build-up in the lining.

So the big question is – why use this rather than other types of HRT? It could be good for women who get side effects from the progesterone component of HRT, such as greasy skin or weight gain. But I think the real benefits will be for women who have low bone density, and want HRT not only to stop menopausal symptoms but also to help prevent osteoporosis.

Bazedoxifene is similar to the drug raloxifene, which is a treatment for osteoporosis. The problem with raloxifene is that it can cause hot flushes and sweats, so it's generally not very popular. But that problem is solved in Duavive because it also contains oestrogen. As yet, there are no trials showing that bazedoxifene on its own can help with bone density, but theoretically the combination could be better for bones than oestrogen alone.

AGE AND HRT

One thing that's very important is all the research on the risks of HRT that has been done on women who are over 50. Some of it has been done on women who are much older – in their sixties. We just don't know the risks of starting HRT before the age of 50, and after all, most women under 50 still have functioning ovaries and their own oestrogen; well, some oestrogen, it may vary a lot from day to day.

I know many experts who say if you have your menopause at 47 or 48 it's possible your risk of breast cancer is slightly lower than your contemporaries – as you have lost your oestrogen – and that taking HRT brings it back up to the normal level. I can't find any good research on this, but I think it's reasonable to assume that taking HRT before 50 is not going to add significantly to your risk of breast cancer. And if you add back the oestrogen you've lost via your skin (using gel or patches) there is certainly no increased risk of a DVT or a stroke.

Women who've had a premature menopause – before the age of 45 – are a different case. This is discussed in more detail on page 19.

OTHER HORMONES – PROGESTERONE AND TESTOSTERONE

The ovaries don't just produce oestrogen, they also produce progesterone and testosterone. There is some evidence that progesterone alone can help reduce flushes and sweats, so it could be an option for women who cannot take oestrogen because of a history of a previous DVT, or those known to be at increased risk of a clot. It is also an option for women who have flushes and sweats and get unacceptable side effects from oestrogen. There is some evidence that micronized progesterone, which is chemically similar to natural progesterone, may have fewer side effects than synthetic progestins, but because it is considerably more expensive it is not widely available on the NHS. Some types of progestogen, such as megestrol, may also be suitable for some women with breast cancer who cannot take oestrogen and who have disabling hot flushes.

Progesterone can also be administered via cream, but in the UK these are only available on prescription. The creams available are unlicensed, which means they have not been approved by the regulatory authorities, and their quality and ingredients cannot be assured. This means that they are not available on the NHS and can only be obtained with a private prescription. Because they are unlicensed, the prescribing doctor has to take responsibility for any effects of the drug, including harmful ones, and because of this very few doctors, especially GPs, are willing to prescribe progesterone creams. There are a few specialists who will prescribe them, but that means paying for a consultation as well as the prescription.

... and testosterone

After the ovaries stop working at the menopause, circulating testosterone levels drop by 50 per cent. Testosterone is known to play a part in libido, and there have also been studies that suggest it has a role in mood and wellbeing. It can also play a role in helping to maintain muscle strength. For these reasons, there has been interest in the use of testosterone in post-menopausal women, especially to help boost sex drive. It was available as a special patch for women, but demand was so low that it's been withdrawn. The only officially licensed form of testosterone now available for women in the UK is in the form of an implant, which is inserted under the skin and needs replacing approximately every six months. It's generally not offered on its own but alongside oestrogen therapy, and generally the implants are only inserted by gynaecologists, not by GPs. Testosterone gel, applied to the skin, is available for men, and theoretically women could use a small amount, but again this is only prescribed and done under specialist supervision.

Side effects of testosterone can occur and can include greasy skin and acne, and an increase in facial hair. These are partly balanced by oestrogen, which is why testosterone is not used on its own. Changes in liver function can also occur, so any women on treatment should have an annual blood test to check liver enzyme levels. Testosterone levels should also be monitored by annual blood tests.

What about bio-identical hormones?

In recent years there seems to have been an increased awareness and demand for 'bio-identical' hormone treatment. Many women seem to perceive bio-identical as meaning 'natural', and that this suggests it is safer and better.

Bio-identical actually means that a hormone is identical in structure to the one made by the body. They are not found in this form in nature, but in fact are manufactured in laboratories. Bio-identical oestrogens are made from yam and soya and include

17-beta-oestradiol, estrone and estriol, and they are found in several standard HRT preparations where the hormones are absorbed through the skin, and also in oestrogen treatments given via the vagina.

More problematic is bio-identical progesterone. The only progesterone available in the UK for use with HRT that is identical to the one made by the body is Utrogestan. This is available in capsule form on the NHS.

Several different 'bio-identical' progesterone creams claim that they can help relieve menopausal flushes and sweats, ease depression and even increase bone density. None of these are currently licensed for use in the UK. There is currently no good solid research from randomised controlled trials and in fact it is possible that not enough active ingredient is absorbed through the skin to make a real difference to any symptoms. This does not really matter if women who buy the cream use it as a sole treatment, and for some just the placebo effect – the belief that they are using something that helps them – may be enough to help relieve symptoms. But it is very important that they are not used as a means of protecting the womb lining in women who are having systematic oestrogen therapy.

It is also important to remember that any medicine (and that includes creams claiming to contain active hormone ingredients) that is not licensed in the UK has no guarantee of safety – either about the way it was manufactured or about its effects in the body.

So that's the basic information. Here are some case histories to illustrate how different forms of HRT suit different women.

Bella, age 48

HER STORY: My periods stopped a few months ago and I'm having the most terrible flushes and sweats. The nights are the worst – I wake up, feel hot, throw the duvet off, and then wake half an hour later freezing cold. I lose count of the number of times this happens, and I'm losing so much sleep I feel exhausted. I work as an accountant, and have to have my wits about me. I think I need HRT, but really don't know much about it. What is it, what are the advantages, and the risks? Will it make me feel normal again, and how long will it take? What type should I take? I hear there are loads of different varieties? What about my periods? A friend told me HRT means they will start again, which I don't mind as long as they aren't heavy.

MY ADVICE: Bella was a good candidate for HRT if she could adjust her lifestyle slightly. She was only 48, and her flushes and sweats were so disabling that she couldn't function properly at work. There was no breast cancer in her family, and I also checked that there was no history of any other significant illnesses either. She admitted she liked a couple of glasses of wine each night (at least) and that would increase her risk of breast cancer. Taking HRT would increase her risk even more – but the greater risk came from the booze. Her blood pressure was normal.

I discussed the various options with her and she decided to start on a low dose of oestrogen gel, one blob a day, and we agreed that if, after a month, she was still having an awful time, she could increase this to two blobs daily. To protect her womb lining, I prescribed her micronized progesterone tablets, to be taken daily for two weeks each month. I warned her that a day or two after stopping these she would have a 'withdrawal' bleed, but, especially on the low dose of oestrogen, this should be quite light.

Zoe, age 51

HER STORY: My last period was about a year ago. I've been having some flushes and sweats, but it's my moods that are the worst problem. I'm really irritable and I'm aware that I'm more anxious than I used to be. I worry about the most stupid things, which is unusual for me. I'm aware I'm not sleeping well, but I'm honestly not sure whether it's because of the flushes and sweats, or because I'm worrying about something silly. My mother has just developed Alzheimer's and has heart disease – and I don't want to go the same way, so would HRT help me? I just want to be back to my old self.

MY ADVICE: Though HRT would help with her flushes and sweats, and also probably even out her moods a little, taking an SSRI or SNRI antidepressant would probably be a better option for her. These are far more effective at levelling out the mood swings and anxiety that can occur at the menopause, and would probably also help with her flushes and sweats. HRT wouldn't make any significant difference to her risk of either heart disease or Alzheimer's – general lifestyle measures (such as losing weight, a healthy diet, lots of exercise and not smoking) are the important things for this. (There is lots more information about antidepressants for treating menopause symptoms in Chapter 4.)

Angie, age 50

HER STORY: My periods have been really erratic for the last six months. I never know when I'm going to have one, and when I do bleed, it's incredibly heavy. I'm also getting some flushes and sweats, which on their own wouldn't be too bad, but every time I get one I feel a bit dizzy and sick beforehand. I have to sit down, which is pretty embarrassing at work, as I'm a retail manager. Would HRT help? Would it control my periods? I'm feeling quite tired and I wonder if all this heavy bleeding has made me anaemic?

MY ADVICE: HRT would help with her flushes, and also help to stop the dizziness and nausea. Her heavy periods were probably just due to fluctuating hormone levels, but before starting HRT I did a pelvic examination to check that her womb was not enlarged. If I had felt anything abnormal, I would have arranged for her to have a pelvic scan. She also needed a blood test to check that she was not anaemic, plus a thyroid function test, as low thyroid hormone levels can cause heavy periods and tiredness. I advised her that the best option for her would be to start with low-dose oestrogen, and she decided to take this in the form of a pill, which she thought would be easier than using gel or patches. I advised her to take the progesterone component in the form of a Mirena; this would thin the womb lining, so hopefully stop the heavy bleeding.

ANGIE, THREE YEARS ON: 'I've been on HRT for three years now and it's really helped the flushes and sweats. You told me the tablets I'm on are a low dose, but I'm really struggling with my weight – I'm up to a size 16 now, and no matter what I do, I can't seem to shift this horrible mutton top around my middle. What are my options? Would the best solution be to stop HRT, and if I do, will the flushes and sweats return?'

MY ADVICE: Angie was already on the lowest possible dose of tablets. One option was to transfer to gel, where she could use a small amount each day, but I suggested that now she had been on HRT for three years and oestrogen appeared to affect her weight quite a lot, the best thing to do would be to try to stop

HRT. However, I advised her to do this very slowly – stopping suddenly often triggers a return of flushes and sweats as the body has no time to adjust to no oestrogen again. She was taking a 'continuous combined' regime, so I suggested taking them on alternate days for at least a month – longer if she had flushes and sweats. Then to go down to one every three days for another month, then one every four days before stopping entirely.

Nareem, age 49

HER STORY: My periods are becoming a bit erratic and I think I'm menopausal. The flushes and sweats have just started, and though I can cope with them at the moment, I wouldn't want them to get any worse. I'm also worried about osteoporosis, as both my mother and aunt have it, so I know it runs in the family, but my aunt also has had breast cancer. Should I start HRT? What about the risk of breast cancer?

MY ADVICE: Her main concern was her bones, and though HRT could certainly be beneficial for them, she would need a full (rather than a low) dose to maintain them and help prevent osteoporosis. She also had a family history of breast cancer, which meant she was slightly more at risk of this, so HRT should be used with caution, especially at high doses. Her flushes and sweats were not too bad, so for her, I advised against HRT at this time. Instead I suggested she should have a bone density scan, to see if she was already at increased risk of osteoporosis, and gave her advice on maintaining her bones by eating plenty of calcium and taking weight-bearing exercise. There is more about osteoporosis in Chapter 6. I also reassured her that if her flushes or sweats became worse we could revisit the idea of HRT.

Mary, age 49

HER STORY: I started on HRT six months ago. I generally feel loads better, my energy and libido are nearly back to where they were, but the monthly periods are heavy, and quite painful, and my breasts feel tender. I find the tablets really easy to take, and am not keen on the patches or gel you previously suggested, but is there another type of tablet I could try? I want something easy – so tablets in a single packet if possible.

MY ADVICE: Mary was taking tablets containing conjugated oestrogens, with additional progesterone in the form of norgestrel for 12 days each month. I suggested switching the oestrogen component to tablets containing 1mg estradiol, which is a different oestrogen, and then tablets containing the same oestrogen but with additional progesterone in the form of norethisterone 1mg for 12 days. If her periods were still heavy after three months, we could keep the oestrogen the same, but switch the progesterone component to dydrogesterone.

Judy, age 52

HER STORY: I've been on HRT now for over a year. It's been wonderful for my flushes and sweats and it's helped me get back to my old self. I'm still working full time, my parents aren't that well, and my eldest is about to leave for uni, which I know I'll find stressful, so I'd like to continue with it. But is there any way I can get rid of the monthly bleeds? They are such a nuisance, especially at my age.

MY ADVICE: Judy was over 50 and had been on HRT for a year, so she could now be switched to a 'continuous combined' regime, where progesterone is given every day alongside oestrogen.

That way she wouldn't have any withdrawal bleeds, though she might get some erratic bleeding for the first few weeks after the switchover. As she was taking tablets containing estradiol and dydrogesterone, I was able to give her exactly the same hormones, which appeared to suit her well.

So that covers HRT. It's a controversial drug, but my view is that it can be wonderful for women who have severe menopausal symptoms and can give you back a normal life. It does have risks, but in my opinion these aren't nearly as bad as they are often made out to be. But that said, it's not for everyone, and stopping it can be difficult – those horrible flushes and sweats may well come back.

It also can be difficult to find a regime that suits you – and you may need to try several before you find the mix that's right. Having a GP or practice nurse who knows about the different types available can be invaluable, so ask at the surgery reception who is the best person to see. If you are having a tough time, don't be scared of going back, time and time again; getting HRT right should be within the skills of a good GP, but if all else fails, ask if you can be referred to a specialist.

SUMMARY

☐ HRT can be wonderful for women with menopausal symptoms and give you back a normal life, stopping flushes and sweats within days.

☐ It has lots of other benefits, too, including helping to prevent osteoporosis and to stop the mood changes that can occur around the menopause, as well as helping to maintain your libido, and skin and hair quality.

- The main disadvantage of HRT is that it can increase the risk of breast cancer, but for most women this increased risk is very small – drinking 14 units a week of alcohol increases the risk by just as much.

- HRT taken by mouth can also increase, very slightly, the risk of blood clots.

- Other side effects can include bloating, weight gain and headaches. Some women also find they get erratic bleeding on HRT.

- The main hormone in HRT is oestrogen, but this can cause thickening of the lining of the womb and, over time, increase the risk of cancer of the womb. This effect can be counteracted by adding in a second hormone, progesterone.

- There are some women who should not have HRT, such as those who have had breast cancer, or a history of blood clots, and if you have high blood pressure it should be back to a normal level with treatment before you start HRT. But HRT is fine for most women – and it's not the baddy it is often made out to be!

- There are lots of different HRT regimes available, and finding the one that suits you can take time. It's best to try each new method for three months, to give your body time to adapt to it. Don't chop and change too quickly.

- The longer HRT is taken, the greater the beneficial effect on bones, but unfortunately, the risk of breast cancer also rises, especially after 10 years of use.

4

MENOPAUSAL MADNESS

Any woman can suffer from emotional issues at any age, and many do. But the time when they often become really troublesome is the years around the menopause. Those who have had problems in the past with anxiety or depression find that what they thought was under control suddenly reappears, and women who have previously never had any problems with their moods find themselves irritable, angry, anxious or depressed, for no apparent reason other than the menopause.

In this chapter I will describe the symptoms so you can – hopefully – recognise if you are affected, I'll explain why they are so common at this time of life and, most importantly, give information about what you can do to return your wayward malfunctioning brain to its normal self.

Commonly asked questions:

I'm still having periods but am getting really bad PMS – much worse than before. Why is this? What can I do about it?

Premenstrual syndrome is caused by the changing levels of oestrogen and progesterone that occur in the menstrual cycle. Around the time of the menopause, hormone levels can be changing wildly not just from one day to the next, but from hour to hour. So severe PMS is really common in perimenopausal women. A range of treatments is available, from hormones, to antidepressants, and exercise can help, too.

My periods are all over the place and so are my moods. I'm really irritable. Why is this?

There are receptors for the hormones oestrogen and progesterone in the brain, which in turn can affect your mood. So as hormone levels change, so can your moods. But it's important to consider other things as well that might be making you irritable, such as tiredness or stress.

Since my periods stopped I haven't been able to enjoy myself like I did before. Will this get better once my body adjusts to not having any hormones?

The changing hormone levels at the time of the menopause can trigger depression, and sometimes this improves once the hormone levels stabilise at their new low level. But this can take many months, so it's worth considering doing something about it. A variety of treatments are available, such as St John's Wort (see page 106), talking therapies (see page 110) or antidepressants (see page 39). Lifestyle adjustments can help, too – see page 36.

I keep getting really anxious about silly things that I never used to worry about before. Is this because of the menopause, and if so, would HRT help?

Many women find they become more anxious around the time of the menopause. Again, it's the changing levels of hormones and the knock-on effect that this has on the chemicals in the brain that control mood. Yes, HRT can help, but so can other treatments, especially antidepressants, which can help with hot flushes, too.

I'm tired all the time. Is this because of the menopause?

If your sleep is disrupted because of night sweats, you are likely to feel tired. The heavy periods that often occur in the perimenopause are a common cause of iron-deficiency anaemia, which in turn can cause tiredness. But it's important to think of other reasons, too, such as trying to do too much all the time, being stressed and being so busy looking after other people that you never have time for yourself – which in my experience is very common in women around the age of 50.

So next I'll go into a bit more detail about why changes in mood are so common around the time of the menopause.

There is no doubt that some women find the thought that they cannot bear children any more profoundly upsetting. The menopause can be a time when some women feel the very heart of their femininity has been torn away, and not surprisingly this can have a negative effect on their mood and general wellbeing.

External lifestyle pressures are common, too. The menopause often occurs at a time when elderly parents are becoming infirm, coinciding with offspring becoming difficult and having hormonal issues of their own. But, most importantly, there are the effects of oestrogen on the brain. There are numerous oestrogen receptors throughout the brain and by acting on these this powerful hormone can influence not only mood, but also memory and concentration. There are a particularly high number of receptors in an area known as the hippocampus, which has an important role in regulating emotions. Oestrogen can also increase levels of brain neuropeptides, such as serotonin, the chemical messengers that play an important role in controlling mood, appetite and sleep. No wonder that menopausal women get mood disorders.

There are, of course, some lucky women who never get a flush or a sweat and who sail through the menopause with no perceptible change in their emotional wellbeing. But many have a much rougher time.

It would be easy to assume that the variations, and especially the low oestrogen levels, that occur at this time of life would mean that all women 'of a certain age' would suffer from mood swings and depression. But that's not the case. There is huge variability in the way different women respond to changing hormone levels, which is probably partly due to the sensitivity of the brain hormone receptors, and also due to background levels of neuropeptides. If you don't make quite enough serotonin, or if you have enough but it can't bind to the receptors on your brain cells, you will be more prone to anxiety and depression.

Self-help for mood problems

No matter whether you are pre- or post-menopause, there are things that you can do that can help. For some with minor symptoms, it may be all you need to do. For others, the change may only be small, and other treatments may be required, but they are always worth a try.

Diet

Tiredness and tension, and emotional ups and downs, can all be eased a little by stabilising your blood sugar levels. That means eating regularly, every three hours, and concentrating on carbohydrates that will give you sustained energy, such as wholemeal bread, wholewheat pasta and wholewheat cereals. That means not indulging in your craving for chocolate biscuits (or similar) because it will only give you a high, then a plunging low sugar level. Not good. Don't skip meals, either – especially breakfast.

Caffeine, particularly large amounts, can make you irritable and can make tension and anxiety worse, and it can stop you sleeping. Cut it down, but do so slowly to avoid thumping caffeine-withdrawal headaches.

Exercise

Exercise has been scientifically proven to boost mood and help relieve depression, anxiety and stress. It's also been shown to be more effective than many hormone remedies at reducing PMS. Even if you feel tired, do something active, every day if possible, especially in the run-up to a period, if you are still having them, or if you feel you are having a 'moody' day. Aim to do something that makes you slightly puffed, for about half an hour. The more you do, the better you will feel.

Annie, age 45

'My doctor told me the best thing to help with my mood swings was to take more exercise. She also said it would help with the battle I was having with my waistline. Looking at her, with her slim figure, and her top-end high-street clothes, and knowing she only worked part-time, I just wanted to scream, "You've got to be kidding! How on earth am I supposed to find the time? I have three teenage kids, and a job, and don't have anyone to clean the house or do the ironing for me. Just give me some pills!"

I met up with a girlfriend a couple of days later and was having a good bitch about my GP when my friend interrupted me, and commented that she was really enjoying the new Zumba class that she was going to on Thursday evenings and why didn't I give it a try? I'd have never done it on my own, but because she was going to be there, I decided I'd give it a go. And you know what? It was really good fun. I felt shattered at the end, and when I got home I was too tired to empty the dishwasher, and told my sons to get off the sofa and do it for me. And for once they did!

So now it's accepted that Thursday evenings are "Mum's time off" for exercise, and the boys make their own supper and clear up afterwards. I think they have sensed that I'm a lot happier after I've done some exercise. So my next target is to add in a second weekly class, and maybe grudgingly admit that my GP may have been talking a bit of sense!'

Practical tips

I'd be the first to admit that fitting a regular exercise regime into your life can be difficult, if not impossible, but it's important to remember that 'exercise' does not have to involve a dedicated session at the gym or doing a fitness session in the local park. Yes, it's great if you can sign up to a weekly class of some sort, and going with a friend can give you an additional impetus to go – especially if you are feeling whacked out after a hard day at work. But if you really can't fit that into your diary, or if you can't find a local exercise class that you want to do, think 'active daily living'.

That means:

- Avoiding escalators and lifts – use stairs instead.

- Rethinking how you get to work. How about walking to / from the station? (Tip – wear trainers and put your heels in your bag.)

- Just because you are approaching 50 does not mean you are too old to get on a bicycle (though I'd admit that helmets aren't great for your blow-dry). And actually when it's not pouring with rain it can often be a really enjoyable way of getting from A to B, and in cities, quicker than using public transport.

- Just because running for the bus has always made you puffed doesn't mean it has to stay that way. Honestly. I know lots of women who used to hate running or jogging who now love it. It's a question of starting really gently, and slowly increasing the amount you do.

- Have a think about how you spend your time after you get home from work. Do you automatically turn on the TV while you empty the dishwasher / load the washing machine? Could it all just wait while you took some time for yourself and went to a yoga or Pilates class? Or even a walk, or a gentle jog? And – challenging thought – would anyone notice, except you?

Sleep

Avoiding becoming overtired is also important. At any time of your life it can make you short-fused, and adding in wayward hormones is just a recipe for a row at home or at work. Make getting enough sleep a priority, along with trying to avoid becoming stressed. If you feel overloaded with things to do, take a couple of minutes to list them in order of priority. Remember, staying sane should be top of the list, and if that means not making the cupcakes you had said you would take to the office, then so be it.

Some recent research has shown that adults need between seven and nine hours a night – and if you get less than that, especially on a regular basis, your health will suffer.

I'm well aware that most women around the age of 50 live frantic lives, usually juggling a job with looking after teenage kids, and often elderly parents as well, but it is really important to make sleep a priority.

It can help to have a good bedtime routine.

- Work out, based on the time you have to get up, when you need to actually get to sleep in order to achieve eight hours of shut-eye.

- Stop whatever you are doing at least half an hour before this time. Turn off whatever screen you are watching, stop ironing or washing up – or whatever else you are doing – and start getting ready for bed.

- If you have been having sweats, or feel a bit sticky, have a shower – it can really help you to sleep better.

- Make sure your bedroom is cool, preferably with some fresh air coming in. At this time of life it can be really helpful!

- Allow yourself some time for relaxation in bed before you turn the lights off – for chatting to your partner, or just some quiet reading.

What about HRT?

If you are approaching the menopause, have erratic periods and are suffering from mood swings, HRT might seem an obvious first choice of treatment. It contains much lower doses of hormones than the combined pill, and this means it doesn't stop your ovaries working but it can add in enough hormones to help even out the wild variations that can occur when the ovaries are winding down in the perimenopause. This in turn can help with PMS and mood swings. However, if your only symptoms are irritability, anxiety or depression, you would probably be better off taking an antidepressant. HRT is a good option if you have other menopausal symptoms and want the additional benefits that HRT can give (and you don't have medical issues that mean it isn't suitable for you). However, getting the 'hormone mix' right can be difficult, especially as some women find that the progesterone component makes a tendency to depression worse. There is more information about this in the HRT chapter on page 73.

MORE DETAILED INFORMATION ABOUT ANXIETY AND DEPRESSION

'I always used to be fairly calm, and it took a lot for me to raise my voice, let alone shout or lose my temper. But when my periods started to become erratic, so did my moods. I lose my rag with the kids over the silliest little things, and I burst into tears a few days ago when I had a really minor prang in the car – so unlike me. I suddenly feel anxious, or just low – and can't enjoy anything any more. I'm just not myself – I just don't know who I am any more.'

No one feels happy and calm all the time, feeling sad, anxious and upset is sometimes quite normal, and is part and parcel of leading a varied life. Life would actually be very boring without a few ups and downs. But you shouldn't feel sad or low most of the time, and neither should you feel constantly worried, or on edge. If you do, you could be suffering from anxiety, or depression, or a mix of the two. These feelings can occur at any age, but women around the age of the menopause are especially at risk.

Being anxious or depressed does not mean you are mad, or inadequate. Both are genuine mental illnesses that are surprisingly common among women, who are affected twice as often as men. However, the gap between the sexes is narrowing a bit, and it may be that women have always been more prepared to admit how awful we really feel compared to men. But there is no doubt that our hormones do us no favours and make us biologically more prone to anxiety and low mood, particularly at times of wild hormonal change, such as after childbirth and around the time of the menopause.

Symptoms

Depression can manifest itself in feelings of emptiness, hopelessness, worthlessness and guilt – that you are not good enough at work, at home, at being a mother, or a friend. You may lose interest in things you once enjoyed, and try as you might, what would previously have given you a buzz, just does nothing, and leaves you flat.

Anxiety makes you fearful and tense. This is a normal reaction if you have something to be afraid of, but it is not when it occurs for no logical reason. In addition to feeling constantly on edge, it's common to have physical symptoms such as palpitations, feeling nauseous and sweating excessively with a dry mouth. Many people with anxiety often get headaches, which are only partly relieved by painkillers.

Sleep disturbance in both anxiety and depression is common, and while some people can't sleep, others – especially those with depression – sleep far more than before, yet still feel perpetually tired. Concentrating and making decisions can be difficult, and you may overeat or starve yourself and never feel hungry. At its worst, feeling anxious all the time can ruin your quality of life, while depression can make you feel as if it just isn't worth living at all.

Why me?

There is no single cause of anxiety or depression. Common triggers for both include an unhappy or abusive childhood, living in a difficult family environment, poverty and stressful events such as losing your job or a relationship break-up. But whereas most people would find this sort of event stressful, then get over it, a person with anxiety or depression finds it impossible to recover back to normality. Chronic illness can also be to blame, especially for depression, along with bereavement, though I'd be the first to admit it can often be difficult to know where normal sadness after losing a loved one turns into clinical depression. And, of course, plummeting oestrogen levels at the time of the menopause can be a major factor. But anxiety and depression can, and often do, occur when there is seemingly no reason at all.

Both anxiety and depression can run in families, and although the common assumption is that this is genetic, in some cases children of anxious or depressed parents receive early lessons in negative thinking.

It's now known that levels of neurotransmitters in the brain, such as serotonin and noradrenaline, can profoundly affect how we process thoughts and how we feel, and that abnormal levels of these can lead to changes in mood, and both anxiety and depression.

As yet, levels of these all-important chemicals can only be assessed using special MRI studies as part of research trials, though I'm sure that one day this will change. What we do know, though, is that some people have inherently low levels of serotonin, and so are more prone to depression, while others have levels that change wildly, causing their moods to alter between deep depression and euphoria. Others appear to have normal brain chemistry until it is altered by an adverse life event.

Both conditions are often diagnosed on just a description of symptoms, but it can be useful to do a formal questionnaire, where you rate a variety of symptoms over the past two weeks. For anxiety, there is a GAD7 questionnaire, while the PHQ-9 is the equivalent for depression. Many GP surgeries have these questionnaires on their website, and these can be useful in determining whether you meet the criteria for a diagnosis of either condition, and also the severity of your illness.

Whatever the cause, both are every bit as genuine an illness as thyroid problems or diabetes, it's just that unlike many other conditions, as yet we can't do a nice easy blood test that confirms that certain chemical levels are not what they should be.

So what can you do about it?

As with all mental illnesses, the first step in the road to recovery is recognising that you have a problem, and to seek help, and that in itself can be a huge hurdle. But being depressed is nothing to be ashamed of, and having it mentioned on your medical records should not affect your ability to get life insurance, or a job.

There are a variety of different treatments, and as with so many conditions, there is no single 'best' treatment. Rather, treatment needs to be tailored to the individual and their symptoms.

Herbal remedies

The best-known herbal remedy for tackling depression is St John's Wort. It has been conclusively proven, in good clinical trials, that it can help to combat mild to moderate depression. However, it is important to take the correct dose, which is 300mcg of the active ingredient hypericin, every day, and also to take it long enough for it to start working. Many mistakenly believe that the herb will make an instantaneous difference to mood, but in fact it takes two to three weeks to make a noticeable difference, and as with all antidepressants, it doesn't work for everyone.

It is also important to be aware that St John's Wort can interact with other drugs, especially the contraceptive pill, and it should not be taken with other antidepressants. Registered St John's Wort products will have a detailed information leaflet in the pack – read it before you start taking it. It can be a good place to start if you want something to lift your mood and for whatever reason do not want to go down the prescription antidepressant route.

Valerian is a traditional herbal remedy that has a sedative action, and there is some evidence that it can help with sleeping problems. It is often also promoted as helping to relieve anxiety and stress, though evidence for this is very limited. Like all medicines that promote sleep, it can make you feel sluggish in the morning, especially at higher doses. Its effects are increased by alcohol and any other medicines that cause drowsiness.

Antidepressants

'I was alarmed – and frightened – when my GP suggested I take antidepressants. I thought they were addictive, and that once I started them I'd never be able to stop, and that they would alter my personality in some way. I also thought that they were really powerful, but my doctor patiently explained to me that they came in various dose levels – and even showed me the list on her prescribing screen – which I found reassuring. And it was silly really, I'd taken St John's Wort without a second thought, believing that because it was "natural" it would somehow be milder than a low-dose antidepressant. But that hadn't helped, and I needed something to manage my anxiety, and also my mood – I constantly felt low, had no energy and found doing anything a real struggle.

For the first few days on the tablets I felt more anxious – but I had been warned about that – and found it difficult to sleep. I also felt a bit sick and generally a bit odd. I was on the verge of giving up, but my partner, who had been really supportive, persuaded me to keep going with them, and by the second week I was sleeping better and my anxiety wasn't so bad. I reckon it took about a month for them to really work properly, and now I really do feel as if I can cope with life's ups and downs, and am enjoying my hobbies again. For me, it was definitely the right thing to do.'

Somehow, antidepressants have become one of those groups of drugs (along with the contraceptive pill and HRT) that some parts of the media love to hate – which of course means that many of the public hate them, too. However, there is really good evidence that they can be very helpful in lifting mood, reducing anxiety and making life more enjoyable again.

There are three main types of antidepressants prescribed by doctors – SSRIs, SNRIs and tricyclics. Whichever you take, it is important to note that antidepressants are not addictive, unlike, for example, alcohol or a tranquilliser, like diazepam, they do not give any immediate effect on mood, so there is no compulsion to take another dose. Neither are there usually any immediate withdrawal symptoms, though, that said, if stopped suddenly they can cause dizziness and electric-shock sensations, which can be worse with SSRIs and SNRIs. For this reason, all antidepressants should be stopped gradually, over a few weeks.

SSRIs, which stands for Selective Serotonin Reuptake Inhibitors, include fluoxetine, citalopram and sertraline. They are the most commonly prescribed group of drugs for anxiety and depression. As their name suggests, they work by preventing the reuptake of serotonin in brain cells, which means it hangs around on the serotonin receptors for longer. In other words, they boost serotonin activity, and this in turn can help alleviate both depression and anxiety. However, they can make anxiety worse in the first few days of treatment, and all patients starting them should be warned of this.

SSRIs usually start to take effect in about a week, but they can take up to three weeks to reach full effect. It's normal to start with a low dose and gradually work up to one where your mood has improved.

Side effects can include a dry mouth, nausea, loose stools and sleep disruption – some find it harder to get to sleep, especially when they first start taking them, while others find they feel sleepy in the middle of the day. More vivid dreams are also reported.

There have also been reports that SSRIs can, very rarely, trigger suicide. The exact reason for this remains unclear, but it may well be that in someone who is severely depressed the drug brings a slight improvement in energy levels and gives them the will to end their life. Whatever the reason, anyone starting treatment should tell someone close to them, especially if they are severely affected.

SNRIs, which stands for Serotonin and Noradrenalin Reuptake Inhibitors, are selective reuptake inhibitors of serotonin and noradrenaline. They include venlafaxine and duloxetine. Unlike SSRIs, they also boost the activity of the brain chemical noradrenaline, and this can be advantageous in those who find SSRIs unhelpful. Like SSRIs, they take time to work and can cause increased anxiety in the first few days of treatment. Side effects can include nausea, a dry mouth, dizziness, tiredness and also loss of appetite. There is also a slightly increased risk of an erratic heartbeat occurring, as well as symptoms on withdrawal, especially when they are used in high doses (which is why they are not usually a first-choice option).

Mirtazapine (an NaSSA) also increases noradrenaline and serotonin activity, but in a slightly different way.

Tricyclics, such as dothiepin and amitriptyline, have a sedative effect and so are suitable for people who have very disturbed sleep. They can cause a dry mouth and constipation, and taking an overdose is more dangerous than with SSRIs. They also take at least three weeks to reach their full effect and are generally only used when other antidepressants don't work. Amitriptyline especially is now used far more for treating chronic pain than for anxiety and depression.

Which one? And how long do you take them for?

As with so many things, there is no 'best' drug – the choice depends on individual symptoms. An antidepressant that suits one person may not suit another. The most popular ones that doctors prescribe are citalopram and fluoxetine. Citalopram has the advantage that it comes in a low-dose – 10mg – tablet, which is often enough for women with mood problems that are not severe. The starting dose for fluoxetine is 20mg, and in smaller women in particular this can cause quite marked side effects, especially to begin with. Fluoxetine lasts longer in the body, though, and this has the advantage that withdrawal symptoms are less likely if you accidentally miss a couple of capsules.

Research suggests that SNRIs are better at controlling hot flushes and sweats than SSRIs. They are therefore often a good choice for women who are having bad physical menopausal symptoms along with mood changes. Venlafaxine is available in a low-dose tablet, 37.5mg, and this may be all that is required to take the edge off symptoms and boost mood. However, side effects can be more problematic than with SSRIs.

The biggest mistake people make with antidepressants is stopping them too soon, the moment they feel better. Instead, they should be continued for at least three months after you feel back to normal. Some people feel remarkably better on them and are able to stop treatment after six months or so, while others need them for much longer. There is no harm in this – everyone's brain chemistry is different.

Talking therapies

There is a bewildering array of different types of talking therapy available, and it can be difficult to know which approach to choose, especially if your mind is foggy or you are constantly anxious. Though you can take yourself off to see a private therapist without a referral, I think it best, if possible, to get guidance from your doctor on the type of treatment that is most likely to be of benefit to you.

There are two main types: counselling and psychotherapy. There is a large overlap between the two, and a lot of counsellors employ some psychotherapy techniques. But putting it very simply, counselling focuses on you talking and thinking your way through a problem, while psychotherapy works on a deeper level, helping you to understand your problems better and to alter the way you think and feel. Neither is a magic bullet, and neither can they alter external pressure in your life, but both can be incredibly helpful and can be used to treat both anxiety and depression, either on their own, or together with antidepressants.

Counselling can alter how you perceive and react to events, and a skilled counsellor can provide objectivity, perception and empathy to give you insight into your behaviour patterns. This in turn can give you strategies for coping with life in a different way, empowering you with choices, whereas before you might have felt the powerless victim. It can enable you to think about a problem in a way that may never have occurred to you before, which in itself can be liberating. Equally importantly, it gives you the freedom to sound off about anything, slag off anyone or burst into tears in complete confidence and without fear of being judged.

Psychotherapy is usually more structured than counselling, and psychotherapists have done a lot more training than counsellors. There are lots of different types of psychotherapy. Some are based around analysing your past life to help you understand why you think and behave as you do – psychoanalysis. Others are based more in the here and now and centre on making you recognise and alter abnormal, dysfunctional thought patterns – cognitive behavioural therapy, or CBT.

Impressive results can often be obtained in just six or eight sessions of CBT, whereas psychoanalysis can take much longer, and this is one of the reasons why CBT is the most common form of psychotherapy available on the NHS. However, if it does not help you, you may be referred for more in-depth psychoanalysis. If you are paying for treatment, discuss with your GP which type of treatment is most likely to be helpful to you.

Severe depression is usually best treated under the care of a psychiatrist. Treatment usually consists of a combination of antidepressants and intense therapy. There is an overlap between psychiatry and clinical psychology, but whereas a psychiatrist is a trained medical doctor, and therefore able to prescribe drugs, a psychologist needs no medical qualification to practise. This means psychologists do not prescribe drugs (unless they have a medical qualification as well).

PMS AND THE PERIMENOPAUSE

It's rare to find a woman who says she has never suffered from PMS. Sometimes it starts in the teenage years, while others find it becomes noticeable after the birth of their first child. But the time it often becomes really severe is when hormones are fluctuating wildly in the perimenopausal years.

There are more than 150 identified symptoms of PMS, ranging from mental ones, such as mood swings, aggression and tearfulness, to physical ones, such as painful breasts, fluid retention and raging headaches. Symptoms vary enormously between individuals, and also from month to month in the same women, especially in the perimenopause.

The symptoms of PMS are thought to be caused by the changing hormone levels. After ovulation, during the two weeks prior to a period, progesterone levels should be about twenty times higher than oestrogen, but commonly, especially in the perimenopause, the gap between the two either widens or narrows, throwing your body out of kilter.

By definition, PMS only occurs in the two weeks leading up to a period, so it's important to keep a mood diary to see if there is a correlation between your emotions and your menstrual cycle. Some women also get symptoms for a couple of days around ovulation, when hormone levels are changing very rapidly. If you have symptoms at other times – for example, in the week after a period – you can't blame PMS for how you feel. This is important in younger women, who may prefer to say they are suffering from PMS when in fact they have clinical depression, or chronic anxiety, in which case treatments for PMS may be inappropriate.

But in the perimenopause, when hormones are all over the place, it's often impossible to know whether it is true PMS or not. This doesn't really matter, as the treatments for true PMS and perimenopausal mood swings are the same.

Getting help from your doctor

There are various treatments available on prescription that can help to ease PMS. Some of these can also be useful in the perimenopause when general hormonal chaos is adding to mood swings.

On the basis that PMS is due to a hormone imbalance, progesterone supplements used to be a very popular remedy. Sadly, though, there is no evidence that this works, and it is no longer recommended.

What can help, though, is switching off the menstrual cycle and so stopping the fluctuating hormone levels that cause PMS. The easiest way of doing this is with the combined contraceptive pill. HRT may also help (see the section below), but it does not override the cycle in the same way.

Danazol and bromocriptine can reduce fluctuating hormone levels and are particularly good for cyclical breast tenderness.

SSRI antidepressants have been shown in numerous clinical trials to be effective at treating PMS. To some, especially those who say that they are not depressed, this can seem like taking a sledgehammer to crack a nut. But the fact is, they work, and around the time of the menopause they can also help to stop flushes and sweats. I'm aware that many women are reluctant to take them, but if your life, and that of your family, is wretched for two weeks before each period, or your erratic hormone levels mean that your moods are constantly up and down, I think they are worth a try. There is more information about these on page 106.

Alternative remedies for PMS

A wide range of supplements are available that claim to relieve PMS symptoms. Unfortunately, there is precious little proper scientific evidence to confirm that they work, but even so, some women have found some of them helpful. Remember, though, that just because something worked well for your best friend does not mean it will work for you, so please don't spend a fortune on a large amount of anything until you have given it a short trial first. For information on alternative remedies for other menopausal symptoms, such as flushes and sweats, see Chapter 2.

Agnus castus contains steroid hormone precursors as well as flavonoids. It is thought that it may have an effect on the pituitary gland via altering the levels of the hormone prolactin. It's been used for centuries to balance female hormones, and there is some good research showing that in some women it can help to alleviate anxiety, fatigue, breast tenderness and bloating linked to changing hormone levels. It is my top recommendation for perimenopausal women troubled by mood swings or PMS.

Wild yam contains both natural plant oestrogens and phyto-progesterone, a natural form of progesterone. Natural progesterone is broken down by enzymes in the stomach, so how much of the hormones in wild yam are actually absorbed into the bloodstream is very questionable. That said, some women say they find it helpful if taken in the couple of weeks before a period.

Dong quai (Chinese angelica root) also has natural oestrogen properties and so may help to balance hormone levels. But beware if your periods are heavy – it could make them worse.

Evening primrose oil is often the remedy quoted as helping PMS, and is often recommended for abdominal swelling and breast discomfort. It contains gamma linoleic acid (GLA) and the suggested dose is 1,000mg a day. However, its official licence for treating breast tenderness was withdrawn because of lack of evidence. If you want to try GLA, I'd suggest you take starflower oil, which contains twice the amount of GLA as evening primrose oil.

Vitamin B complex (particularly with added magnesium and chromium) has been claimed to relieve sugar cravings, irritability and bloating. Vitamin B6 is particularly popular, but don't exceed the recommended dose because it can damage the nervous system. Try 100 to 400mg daily, beginning around 10 days before your period is due. Don't take this amount all the time, though.

STRESS

Lisa, age 48

'I had always thought I was one of life's "copers" – and I knew everyone regarded me as the walking example of "ask a busy person if you want something done". I'd always worked ever since I left university, and took very little time off from my job as an NHS manager when I had my three kids. I was on the PTA committee, and would be the first to volunteer when someone was needed for a fete, or to make cakes. But then my mum, who lived a three-hour drive away, was diagnosed with breast cancer, and needed help after her mastectomy and through her chemo. At the same time, we had a big inspection coming up at work, and my deputy manager resigned as her partner's job had moved. I found myself trying to fill in spreadsheets at midnight, after I'd driven back from Mum's, and when I did eventually get to bed, I couldn't sleep. I found myself snapping at the kids, and completely forgot to go to a parents' evening at my daughter's school. She was so upset, and I was mortified. I realised I just couldn't manage any more and went to my GP, as I thought I was having some sort of breakdown. She explained I was just very stressed and needed some time away from the pressures of work, and that I needed to stop trying to be superwoman and learn to say no.'

We all benefit from a little stress – without it life can seem very dull – and there is evidence that lack of stress can be a factor in depression. Stress stimulates the body's fight or flight response, and helps us to think and react faster, giving us the buzz that helps us through the marathon of childbirth, or meeting an impossible deadline at work, and managing to get to a parent–teacher meeting at the end of a long day.

But too much stress is a different thing altogether. It makes us feel out of control, exhausts the immune system and opens the door to mental and physical illness. And many women today experience intense stress because of the twin demands of home and work, and because they spend a disproportionate amount of time and energy caring for others at the expense of their own needs and wellbeing.

So what are the signs of stress?

Some people know when they are stressed, but I've seen lots of people who are unaware of it. It has become such a 'normal' part of their day-to-day life that they don't realise that the irritability at work, difficulty getting to sleep and inability to relax are all because their mind – and often their body as well – is simply overloaded.

When you are stressed out your behaviour is likely to affect those around you, as you tend to appear to be spoiling for a fight, whether it is with family or work colleagues. Sometimes the aggression is verbal, but it can also spill over into road rage (yes, women get it too) or physical violence. Physical symptoms can include constant headaches, chest pains, palpitations and skin problems.

Though there is no doubt that overwork and trying to do too much can be very stressful, how you react to adverse events can make a difference to your stress levels. If, for instance, your train to work is cancelled, a calm person will phone the office, explain it's out of their control, and settle down to read another chapter of their book. In contrast the stressed-out person will let out a stream of abuse about the state of the railways to anyone in earshot and pace the platform like a caged lion.

If any of this sounds familiar, your life probably needs a rethink. You need to regain control, know your enemy and identify situations that trigger feelings of powerlessness, panic and anger. Even if you can't avoid stressful situations (and I'm well aware that a lot of women can't), you need to make a determined effort to alter how you react to them.

Self-help for stress

Stress management takes time and practice, and it starts with the recognition that you are not – and nor should you want to be – superwoman. This means:

- Learning to say 'no', and delegating tasks to others. You do not have to do everything yourself. Your family would prefer you to serve up a ready meal than be tearing your hair out and shouting at them while slaving over a hot stove at the end of a long day at work.

- Making more time for yourself and spending it doing things that give you pleasure. It really is OK to be selfish sometimes – it's called 'self-preservation'.

- Take exercise, listen to music that you enjoy (even if others can't stand it!), eat a healthy diet and don't try to blot out your feelings with alcohol or drugs.

- Have realistic expectations of what you can achieve in a day. Forward planning can do a lot to minimise stress. Allow yourself plenty of time to do tasks, because being late or chasing the clock will put you under pressure. Operate a strict priority system to minimise your load – some things really can wait.

Over half of all illnesses are now reckoned to be stress-related, ranging from recurrent coughs and colds through to high blood pressure, strokes and heart attacks. If you have tried to make your life more manageable but still feel like running away or quitting your job, or are constantly shouting at those around you, see your GP. Explain honestly what has been happening and discuss with your doctor what treatment, or therapy, would be of most help to you.

HEADACHES AND MIGRAINES

Headaches have to be one of the most common health problems in women. Like many other ailments, they can occur at any age, but they often become more noticeable around the time of the menopause. Not only can changing hormone levels trigger headaches in their own right, but they can also influence other factors that can cause headaches, especially tension and stress.

Tension headache is the most common form of headache that I see in my surgery. It is caused by tightening of the muscles of the scalp, but the pain is often felt across or behind the eyes, across the forehead or sometimes right inside the skull. Tension headaches are often linked to anxiety and stress. They can also be caused by a stiff, tender neck, which may in itself be a sign of stress or be due to mild arthritis. Tension headaches may only occur occasionally, but in some women they can become a daily problem that starts on waking.

Analgesic abuse headache is another common cause of headache. Abuse here doesn't mean addiction, it just means taking too many ordinary painkillers, such as ibuprofen or paracetamol, on a regular basis. The brain gets used to them and doesn't like it when it has to do without. Keep a note of how many painkillers you are taking. If it's more than 30 a month and you are getting frequent headaches, the pills could be to blame. Cutting down can be difficult, as the headaches often get worse, and you may need the help of alternative types of pain-modifying drugs, such as amitriptyline (available on prescription from your GP).

Hunger, dehydration (particularly when it's caused by an excess of alcohol) and a sudden drop in caffeine intake can also cause headaches. If you are cutting down on caffeine, always do it slowly.

Headaches can also be caused by eye strain, and remember that around the time of the menopause your sight will be changing, and you are likely to need reading glasses, and maybe a separate pair for use on a computer.

Though many people worry about headaches, on their own they are rarely a sign of anything serious. It's when a blinding headache is accompanied by vomiting, dizziness or feeling disorientated that you need to worry and hotfoot it to your doctor. But if you suddenly start getting headaches for no obvious reason, you should also go and see your GP.

Migraines are no ordinary headaches. A migraine is a severe thumping headache that usually, but not always, is felt on one side of the head, often preceded by an 'aura' which may be flashing lights, a strange smell, nausea or vomiting.

The exact cause for migraines isn't known, but it is thought that they are linked to changes in the blood vessels inside the brain, triggered by a small change in serotonin activity. They are much more common in women, and tend to occur when hormone levels are changing rapidly. That means they often occur around the time of a period, and become more frequent, and unpredictable, around the time of the menopause. Thankfully, once hormone levels are settled after the menopause they usually become less frequent.

HRT can be helpful during the transition – but not always, as in some it can make migraines worse.

There is increasing evidence that drugs used to treat chronic pain, such as pregabalin or gabapentin, may help prevent migraines, and these can be particularly useful when your hormones are completely out of kilter. Unlike other types of painkillers, they don't work straight away but must be taken for several weeks, at a slowly increasing dose.

Pam, age 48

HER STORY: I've not been myself for a while. I've noticed I've been really short-fused with the family, and last weekend I really lost my rag and threw a box of cornflakes across the kitchen. They went everywhere. The kids were really shocked, and my husband was appalled. I don't think he can take much more.

My periods are slightly more frequent than they used to be, but still regular, but I have noticed I'm much more moody in the week before each one. I'm always tired, though – I've got so much on my plate – what with trying to run my own business, and then when I get home I often have to collect the kids from after-school activities, get their dinner and get the washing in. And then at weekends I have to go and see my father, who has recently had a stroke – it's a 400-mile round trip. So I never get a chance to sit down. I don't see what can alter with my lifestyle but I was wondering if there was anything that could help with my terrible mood swings. A friend recommended agnus castus from the health-food shop, as she said it helped her, but to be honest, I didn't notice any difference. At my age, would HRT be any good?

MY ADVICE: Pam was a classic case of a woman in her late forties with severe premenstrual syndrome. Her lifestyle wasn't helping, and one of the first things she needed to do was take steps to reduce her stress levels and try to get more sleep – easier said than done, though. (There is more about this on page 101.) I explained that HRT might help her, as could the combined contraceptive pill, which would be suitable for her as she was otherwise healthy, didn't smoke, and wasn't overweight. I then gave her the option of antidepressants. She then admitted that in fact she often felt irritable in the weeks after her period, and maybe everything that she was trying to cope with was getting her down and that she might be mildly depressed, as well as having severe PMS. I prescribed her a low dose of citalopram, an SSRI antidepressant. I advised her not to start it while she was in her premenstrual week, as initially it can make anxiety worse – which might be a recipe for another packet of thrown cornflakes. Instead she started it immediately after her period, and though she did initially have some problems with nausea and a dry mouth, these side effects eased after the first week, and she gradually began to feel much better. Six months on, she says she is still a bit moody but in an unpredictable way as her periods have now become irregular. If her symptoms become worse as her menopause approaches, switching, or adding in, HRT is an option.

Jayne, age 50

HER STORY: I need some advice about the menopause. I just haven't got any energy. I'm constantly tired and just have no will to go out – and when I do I don't really enjoy myself. I also often feel really anxious, to the point where I can't function. My daughter recently passed her driving test and I've been convinced that she is going to have a terrible accident. I know every parent worries when their kids start driving, but the thought of her being killed on a motorway is going round and round in my head, and it stops me sleeping at night – which I'm sure is why I'm so tired. My last period was about six months ago. I haven't had much in the way of flushes or sweats, but I wonder if I need HRT? I need to do something to sort myself out.

MY ADVICE: Jayne was clearly suffering from anxiety, and her lack of energy and inability to enjoy herself suggested she was depressed as well. This was confirmed when I asked her some more questions about her general mood and her appetite, which was poor. I discovered she had been feeling more anxious than usual for several years, but it had become much worse around the time of the menopause. Though HRT would probably help a little, I advised that the best treatment for her would be cognitive behavioural therapy, which could help her tackle her irrational thoughts. I also suggested that antidepressants might help, too, but she wasn't keen on taking these, preferring something she felt was more natural. I suggested St John's Wort, and also taking regular exercise to try to boost her mood. Three months on she had started both St John's Wort and her CBT sessions and said she felt a little better, though she was still anxious when her daughter borrowed her car. She said the thing that helped most, though, was her weekly spinning class. I saw her again a few months later, after she had completed her CBT. She told me she had found the sessions quite hard, and challenging, and had discovered she was irrational and anxious about lots of things – and probably always had been – but at least now she could recognise when she was thinking in a negative way and try to put a positive slant to her thoughts.

Mary, age 52

HER STORY: My best friend said I should come and see you, but I'm not sure if you can really help. My marriage has been bad for ages – my husband has had several affairs, but he's always apologised afterwards and said he doesn't want our marriage to end. I threatened to leave him a couple of years ago, so he promised he would be faithful. Then around six months ago I found another load of sexy texts on his phone, and we had a blazing row. I'd already moved into the spare room – with all the hot flushes I've been having it actually suited me better to sleep with the window wide open, but he complained he felt cold. I wish I had the courage to leave him, but I don't. Who else is going to want me at my age? Since my periods stopped I feel I'm not attractive any more, and that I've well and truly hit middle age. I don't have any energy to do anything, and I feel exhausted from the moment I wake up until the time I try to go to sleep, though the flushes keep waking me up. I've been drinking too much as well – drowning my sorrows, I suppose. The kids are off at university, and I don't think anyone would really notice if I wasn't around any more, though I wouldn't do anything silly, as it would upset them too much. But it has crossed my mind. I feel so pathetic.

MY ADVICE: It was obvious from what she had said that Mary was suffering from low mood, so I went through a PHQ-9 questionnaire with her. She scored 19 out of 27, confirming that she had severe depression. I suspected that she had been depressed for several years, and that the menopause and her husband's behaviour had recently made it more severe. Her ongoing tiredness, caused by flushes disrupting her sleep, wasn't helping either. She was also suffering from very low self-esteem, brought on by her husband's repeated affairs, and by the feeling that the menopause meant she wasn't a 'proper woman' any more.

I felt she needed both antidepressants and psychological therapy – I didn't think that either alone would tackle all her issues. I also suggested that if antidepressants didn't help with her hot flushes then she might want to consider HRT to help with those and her sleepless nights. This would be a safe option for her, as she had no family history of breast cancer or of blood clots, and she had no underlying medical problems.

I kept a close eye on her, and saw her every couple of weeks for a few months. The antidepressants did help lift her mood but did nothing for her flushes, so after a month she decided she wanted to try HRT. Because her periods had stopped more than a year ago, she was able to have a continuous combined regime. She wanted tablets, which she said she would find easier than gel or patches, so I gave her a low dose containing 1mg of progestogen. Initially she felt a bit bloated, but within a fortnight her flushes had improved, along with her sleep, and she said she felt much better in herself.

A course of therapy helped improve her self-esteem, but six months on she was still with her husband – who was continuing to make her miserable. So far he has, apparently, refused to go to the marriage guidance counselling. I have no idea how it will end, but there are some issues that doctors just can't solve.

Marie, age 50

HER STORY: I've been getting terrible migraines. I've always tended to have headaches around the time of my period, but now I'm getting them nearly every day. It feels as if there is a tight band around my head. Paracetamol and ibuprofen help, but I'm having to take them several times a day. My periods are still regular, but I wondered if it's the menopause, and if so, what can I do about it?

MY ADVICE: Marie, a single mum, was working long hours running her own internet business, and because she mainly worked from home, she didn't think she could justify having any help looking after her three teenage children. She admitted that life was a juggling act of shopping, cooking, cleaning, acting as a chauffeur for her kids and trying to get to school events. The father of her children had moved 200 miles away, and the kids did go away some weekends to see him, but Marie used this time as an opportunity to concentrate on her work. From what she said, she had no relaxation time at all.

As her periods were still regular it was unlikely that the menopause was to blame in her case. I thought it more likely that she was suffering from a combination of stress-induced headaches which were being made worse by taking daily painkillers.

I advised her that though it was admirable that she was making such an effort to be a supermum, she needed to make looking after herself more of a priority. Her kids were old enough to help out more around the house, and though it would probably be difficult at first, she needed to delegate tasks to them, like doing their own washing and ironing and cooking a meal once a week. This would hopefully give her some time for relaxation and, more importantly, some exercise (which she admitted she had not done since her kids were born). She also needed to wean herself off the daily painkillers.

I checked up on her a couple of months later. She told me she'd had a rough time with the children refusing to help until she had entered for a 10km run to raise money for a local charity. This had given her the impetus to make sure she got time outside the house and for the kids to start lending a hand. The headaches hadn't gone completely, but they were less frequent, and she was only taking paracetamol a couple of times a week. But on the downside, she had missed a couple of periods and was having a few hot sweats. But for the time being she said she didn't want any treatment for them, as they were bearable. But she warned me that if they got any worse, she would be back knocking on my door!

SUMMARY

- Mood changes are very common around the time of the menopause, due to changing hormone levels.

- During the perimenopause, premenstrual syndrome often becomes a lot worse.

- Anxiety and depression are common in women of menopausal age and are often at their worst just after periods stop.

- Women of menopausal age often drive themselves very hard and make everyone else their priority. Not surprisingly, this can lead to stress – which makes anxiety and depression worse.

- Self-help measures – taking more care of yourself, making time for relaxation and exercise and eating a balanced diet – should be top of every woman's list when tackling mental health issues.

- Do not be afraid to speak to your doctor. You will not be labelled as being weak or mad, and the most effective treatments – either tablets, or talking therapy – are usually only accessible via your GP.

- Antidepressants can help relieve both anxiety and depression, and can help with hot flushes as well.

- If you want to avoid antidepressants, herbal remedies, especially St John's Wort, can be helpful in some women.

5

WHAT HAS HAPPENED TO MY WAISTLINE?

It is incredibly rare to find a woman in her fifties who has the same waist measurement as she did in her twenties. Many women assume that it's having babies that changes their shape as they get older, but actually that's a myth. It's true that many women do gain weight during pregnancy, and it does inevitably stretch your abdominal muscles, but it's perfectly possible (if you work hard enough at it) to get back your pre-pregnancy shape and waistline.

However, even the most figure-conscious women notice that in their early fifties their shape changes, with a thickening of their waistline. The culprit, yet again, is the change in hormone levels.

So what I'm going to do in this chapter is explain why your shape changes and, more importantly, what you can do about it!

As before, I'll start with some commonly asked questions and then go on to more detailed background information, and include some case histories.

Trish, age 54

'I always used to be slim, and though I wasn't one of those people who could eat anything and not put on a pound, I didn't feel it was too difficult to stay in shape. If my clothes felt tight I just cut back a bit for a while, and that seemed to do the trick, even after I had my kids. And I felt I looked OK in a bikini, even when I was in my forties. But now I'm 54, my body seems to be completely different. I'm not overweight, but I'm not as slim as I used to be, and I find it really difficult to shed any weight at all. I haven't altered my diet, and I walk the dog every day, but my skin feels flabby, I don't feel I've got any shape – certainly no waist – and I can see horrible little bulges above and below my bra across my back. And there is no way I'd wear a bikini now. I simply don't recognise my own body any more.'

The common questions:

Why has my shape changed? Is it my hormones?

As women grow older it is normal for their fat distribution to change, and for more fat to accumulate in the abdominal area. And as the skin gradually ages, it loses its support, so that firm curves become more, well, flabby. The loss of oestrogen at the menopause accelerates this ageing process, too, which means the time you tend to notice that you are not the shape you once were is in your early fifties.

But what about the weight gain? Why is it so hard to keep the pounds off – and even harder to lose them?

Unfortunately, losing weight really does get harder as you get older, simply because your metabolic rate – the rate at which your body burns calories – slows down with increasing age.

The main reason for this is because of loss of muscle – or sarcopenia, as the medics call it. (There is more information about this on page 135.)

Could it be my thyroid?

The way that weight creeps on for seemingly no reason means that many women feel something medical must be to blame, such as an underactive thyroid. Though it's true that thyroid problems are more common in women than men, and they tend to occur in midlife, the cruel reality is that an underactive thyroid is very rarely to blame for an enlarging waistline around the menopause. In my experience as a GP, women who have an underactive thyroid hardly ever have just weight gain – other problems are much more of an issue for them, such as tiredness, thinning hair or just feeling a bit sluggish.

So what can I do about it?

Once you are in midlife you have to take a two-pronged attack to lose weight: *exercise* and *diet*. Yes, you can lose weight by doing just one of these, but it's far easier to shift that midriff bulge if you do both.

So you're telling me I've got to exercise. What if I've always been a couch potato? Am I going to hurt myself?

You are never too old to start doing exercise. Even if you have always been a couch potato and just the thought of getting hot makes your sweats worse – you can do it. Just start slowly and gradually increase what you do.

It's also good to try to incorporate more activity into your daily life. Just little things, such as taking the stairs instead of an escalator or lift, and walking to the local shops, can make a difference. If exercise could be bottled, it really would be a wonder pill that could keep many illnesses at bay. Trouble is, of course, keeping active takes time and motivation. But at the menopause it really is important to make this a priority.

How much should I weigh?

The aim at this time of life should not be to have a classic hourglass figure or even a flat tummy. What you should be aiming for is to be a healthy weight and shape, so that your risk of arthritis, heart disease and diabetes is low. And if you are at a healthy weight, the chances are you will also have a little fat, which is important at this age. (There is more information about this on page 140.)

But shouldn't I aim to be the weight I was when I was younger?

No, not only is it incredibly hard to try to keep the shape you had when you were in your twenties, but *it's not healthy to do so, either*. There is a biological reason for that 'middle-aged spread'. After the menopause, what little oestrogen your body has comes from the conversion of androgens (produced in the adrenal glands) and this occurs in fat cells. The fewer fat cells you have, the lower your oestrogen levels are going to be. Even having a little oestrogen has health benefits, so you can really be too thin for your own good. Of course, the converse of this is that fatter older women have higher oestrogen levels, and this is thought to be why they are more at risk of both breast and womb cancer. As always, there is a happy medium that all women should strive for, which is good for not only your health but also your looks. The plump cheeks of youth mean that you can get away (just) by being a bit thin but still looking good, but by the time you are approaching 50 people are likely to notice a gaunt face more than a slightly rounded tummy.

GETTING INTO SHAPE

Penny, age 56

'It was the group family photo that did it. I was standing sideways on, and my stomach was sticking out so much I looked pregnant. My posture was awful, and my arms and legs looked flabby. I'd never bothered much about exercise, and couldn't possibly afford to join a gym anyway. But I had to do something. I asked around, and found a Pilates class at my local church hall that was really cheap. I was really scared about going to begin with, as I didn't know anyone. But the teacher was friendly, and I realised as soon as I walked in that there were plenty of other people there who weren't experts and who had the same type of body as me. After the first session I was hurting in places where I didn't know I had muscles, but I really enjoy it now, and my posture and flexibility have definitely improved. I need to do something more energetic to shift the roll of flab around my middle, so I'm going to try out a beginners military fitness class in the local park. I'd have never dared to do this if I hadn't joined the Pilates class, but that has given me the confidence to give new things a try.'

I'm going to start this section with exercise, because I reckon it's the bit that many women tend to push to the back burner. And actually, if you are like most of my patients, and are trying to tackle your waistline, you are probably already on some sort of diet. But chances are, if your diet is not being successful, you are not exercising as much as you should be.

The importance of exercise

In order to lose weight, your body needs to use up more calories than you eat. The bigger the difference, the more weight you will lose. Yes, if you cut right back on your food and don't do any exercise then you will lose weight, but this is bad for two reasons. Firstly, your body will go into 'starvation' mode, and your basal metabolism will fall. Secondly, you will lose muscle as well as fat, pushing your resting metabolism down even further. So when you do start eating again, you'll find you suddenly gain weight, even if you are not eating very much.

Here's where exercise comes in.

First of all, a bit about the different types of exercise.

Cardiovascular exercise (often called cardio for short) pushes up your heart rate and makes you puffed – stuff like jogging, skipping or doing a Zumba or step class.

Then there is *strength training*. This is the type of exercise that helps to maintain muscles. It involves working your muscles against resistance, such as lifting weights, or working machines in a gym.

Both these types of exercise are important in the battle against the midriff bulge, and there's more detail about them in the sections that follow.

Women also need to know about a third type of exercise: *weight-bearing* exercise – which is important for maintaining bones. This is covered on page 163.

So, first …

Cardiovascular exercise

This involves movement that speeds up your heart rate and your breathing rate, so more blood is pumped round the body to deliver oxygen to muscles. Once inside the muscles, that oxygen is used to burn fat and carbohydrates to provide energy to keep them working. Examples of cardio exercise are running, swimming, hiking and aerobics classes. Cardiovascular exercise improves the functioning of the heart – like any other muscle, if it's worked hard it gets stronger and bigger. It's cardio exercise that makes you physically fit and able to walk up a hill, or run up a flight of stairs without becoming out of breath.

Health benefits

The health benefits of cardiovascular exercise are huge, apart from helping with weight control. It helps prevent heart disease, not only by strengthening the heart itself, but also by lowering blood pressure and making blood vessels more elastic and less likely to accumulate fat in their lining. It is key in preventing diabetes not only by helping weight loss, but also by preventing the body becoming resistant to the action of insulin. It has been proven to help prevent both breast and colon cancer, and can help to both prevent and treat depression. It can also help keep your brain functioning well, and rates of dementia are lower in people who take regular exercise.

When you are doing cardiovascular exercise your body burns more calories. Just how many extra depends on your size – the larger you are, the more calories your body needs – and also on the type of exercise you are doing. But in addition, your body continues to burn calories at a higher rate after you have stopped exercising, so the more often you exercise, the higher your metabolism will be.

Did you know?

The more cardio you do, the more you increase small organs inside the muscles' cells, called mitochondria, that are the energy factories that burn oxygen. The more mitochondria you have, the more exercise you are able to do, and the more calories you will burn.

Cardio alone is fine when you are young and have lots of muscle, but by the time you are 50, the chances are you have lost a lot of muscle bulk. You need to do strength training to hang on to what you have, and build some back up again.

So next – strength training.

Strength training

This is the type of exercise that helps to maintain muscles, and is vital in helping to prevent sarcopenia – the loss of muscle that occurs as you get older. The most obvious example of strength-training exercise is anything that involves lifting weights, but anything that repeatedly works a muscle will help to keep it strong, so sit-ups and squats count, too, as does exercise involving pulling large elastic strips. It's strength training that is important for giving you tone and balance, and when you are older, helping to prevent falls. It also helps to keep your arms and legs strong, so you can lift that flat-pack furniture or pile of floor tiles out of the boot of your car without your arms or legs giving way. There is also evidence that any type of strength training can help maintain the strength of the bone to which the muscle is attached – so for instance, lifting weights with your arms will help prevent a wrist fracture, while doing leg-weight work will help prevent a hip fracture.

Health benefits of strength training

From the time you are born to around the age of 30, your muscles grow larger and stronger, but in your fourth decade you begin to lose muscle tissue. People who are physically inactive can lose as much as 5 per cent of their muscle mass per decade after the age of 30, and even if you are reasonably active – going for a weekly run, or a game of tennis – your muscles will still get smaller. It's the muscle equivalent of osteoporosis.

The importance of muscles

Muscle burns more calories than any other type of tissue, and as the quantity of muscle falls, so too does the metabolic rate. Your metabolic rate – the rate your body uses calories at rest – falls by about 3 per cent a year from your mid-thirties, and the main reason for this is loss of muscle. It's why, if you continue to eat at 45 what you ate when you were 25, you will inevitably gain weight. Research has shown that the average woman gains about 4.5kg (10lb) of fat between the ages of 34 and 47, and unfortunately, fat cells, metabolically speaking, are very sluggish – they burn calories at the lowest rate of all the types of body tissue. Pound for pound, muscle burns twice as many calories as fat.

At the age of 30, an average woman needs about 2,000 calories a day, a bit more if she is active. Once you are 51, that's fallen to 1,600 – again, maybe 1,800 if you are reasonably active. No wonder that a standard 1,500-calorie-a-day weight-loss diet doesn't work.

Sarcopenia is just as important as osteoporosis for several reasons. Though it's true that muscles don't break, loss of muscle can be just as devastating for your health as loss of bone.

You need good muscles to keep fit and active, which is incredibly important for your mental and physical health. If you want to be able to go for long walks with your family, or continue playing badminton (and having a hope of beating younger members of your family) you need decent muscles.

Muscles are also vital for giving your body shape and tone, and unless you take action, you are unlikely to maintain reasonably toned arms and legs and your bottom will go flat. The latter may seem appealing, but having no curve at all to your derriere is very ageing. It's not just flushes and sweats that signal you have reached 'a certain point in your life'; your jeans don't look as good as they used to, and you realise that maybe it's time to wear dresses with sleeves.

It's also muscles that hold your joints in place, so if you have weak muscles you are more likely to twist your knee and ankle if you trip on a loose paving stone. Strong muscles help preserve joint stability and reduce the risk of injury; if you have strong muscles, you'll also have better balance, and are less likely to fall over and break your wrist or your hip. Muscles provide vital support for your spine, and having weak back muscles is one of the major contributing factors to back pain.

So if you want to maintain your strength and fitness and control your waistline as you get older, you have to take steps to preserve your muscles. I'm not talking here about becoming a female version of Arnold Schwarzenegger, with bulging thighs and biceps, I'm talking about having toned, firm muscles that give your body shape and allow you to move freely, and without pain.

Working your core

You've probably heard of 'core exercises', but many women I meet don't know exactly what their core is, let alone know how to 'work it'!

135

Your core muscles are the ones that support your body, and though these include the muscles in the back, they are mainly the ones in the front of your abdomen. They play a very important role in supporting your body, and if your core is strong, you are less likely to suffer from back problems. The core muscles also help you to maintain your posture. A woman with a strong core stands straight and can wear a fitted dress without having to resort to uncomfortable support underwear. Having a good core doesn't guarantee you a flat washboard stomach, as your shape will also be dictated by the amount of fat you have, but you will look far less saggy than those with weak core muscles. The most well-known core exercise is doing sit-ups, but they must be done properly – not only to work the muscles, but to avoid putting a strain on your neck and back.

To learn how to do core exercises, I suggest you join a Pilates class or, if you prefer, you can teach yourself in your own home using an instructional video.

So how much exercise do I really need to do?

The best type of exercise for burning calories, and therefore shedding pounds, is cardio stuff. The best 'fat-blasting' exercise should be intense enough to make you hot and sweaty, and a little breathless, and should be sustained for at least 20 minutes (though half an hour is even better) and should be undertaken regularly, ideally three times a week. Luckily, this is also what has been shown to be what's needed for the other health benefits, too. So even if you are not trying to lose weight, you should aim for this amount – you just don't need to cut calories as well!

The trouble is, the energy the body uses for cardio exercise doesn't just come from the fat that you are so keen to get rid of, the body also breaks down muscle. To stop this happening you need to do strength training as well, ideally for at least an hour a week, working on different muscle groups in your body – arms, legs and, most important of all at this age, your bum and your abdominal muscles.

Exercise and weight loss

Vigorous exercise, such as an energetic dance class, or running fast, can increase your metabolic rate by six to ten times the resting rate. A 50-year-old woman weighing 60kg will burn about 50 calories an hour at rest, but going for a fast run for 40 minutes will burn an additional 450 calories. Doing that regularly can make a big difference to your waistline and your thighs.

One study showed that in overweight people who were placed on a calorie-controlled diet and who did regular cardiovascular exercise, 31 per cent of the weight they lost came from muscle. A similar group, who followed the same regime but included some strength training, lost exactly the same overall amount of weight, but only 3 per cent came from muscle.

So that's the exercise bit, but to manage your weight at this time of life you need to take a careful look at what you are eating – and drinking.

DIET

Julia, age 50

'I was invited for an NHS health check at my local surgery, and having just turned 50, I thought it would be a good idea to go along. I knew my weight had crept up a bit, and my size-14 clothes were getting a bit tight, but I thought that was normal for someone of my age. I was shocked when the nurse told me I was so overweight I was borderline medically obese. Worse still, my blood test showed that I was "pre-diabetic", and the only way to stop myself becoming diabetic was to lose weight.

To begin with the nurse suggested I took a photo on my phone of all my meals and drinks – she said it was easier for her to judge portion size that way than if I was writing it down. She said my diet wasn't that unhealthy, but I was just eating too much for a woman of my age. I'd never realised before that you don't need as much food at 50 as you do when you are 20. I realised a crash diet wasn't the answer, and that I needed to change my eating habits, long term, which meant that some of the foods I really liked, such as lasagne and creamy curries, just had to go. I also found it hard to adjust my portion sizes and often felt really hungry. I think what kept me at it was the thought of being diabetic – that really motivated me to get the pounds off.'

Speak to any doctor or dietician and they will tell you that the best way to lose weight is to eat a well-balanced, low-calorie diet, with plenty of fruit and vegetables. The trouble is this can be boring, and it can be quite difficult working out exactly what you can and cannot eat. No wonder a huge multimillion-pound dieting industry has appeared. Someone, somewhere has made a mint out of advising women to trim their figures by eating nothing but cabbage soup or grapefruit, or to cut out carbs completely, or to eat hardly anything for two or three days a week. These sorts of diets may be fine if you have just a few pounds to lose, but if you're looking at getting off more than half a stone, you need a diet you can follow for weeks at a time. Different diets work for different people, and just because a particular diet suits your best friend doesn't mean it will suit you.

To lose 1lb of fat means you have to have a deficit of around 3,500 calories. I usually tell my patients to aim to lose around 1lb – that's around half a kilo – a week. That may not seem very much, but at this rate of loss you should be able to eat a reasonable diet, with occasional treats – in other words, something that you stick to, long term. If you lose more than 2lb a week your body will, to some extent, be going into starvation mode. Unless you are doing a heck of a lot of weight training, you will be losing muscle as well as fat, and the moment you start eating anything resembling a normal diet, the pounds will pile on again.

Whole books have been written on diets, and I haven't got space here to go into detail of what you should and should not be eating, but here are some tips that my patients tell me have been useful.

- Eat only when you are hungry. Eat slowly, and only eat enough to satisfy your hunger. However, be careful; around the time of the menopause many women feel light-headed, get headaches or feel unduly tired if their blood sugar falls a little low. The best way to combat this is to eat little and often, rather than having a once-daily big meal.

- Don't skip meals, especially breakfast. It gives your metabolism a boost at the beginning of the day.

- When you first start dieting, weigh your food so you know what a 'portion' should look like. Switching to smaller plates can be a good way of training yourself to eat less at meals.

- Opt for foods that give sustained energy, such as those made with wholegrains, and avoid sugary snacks which give an instant boost to blood sugar – your blood sugar levels will only plummet soon after, and you'll feel hungry again.

- Watch your alcohol intake. Not only is alcohol full of calories, with no nutritional benefit, but it can wreck your willpower, too.

- Eat plenty of lean protein, such as fish and poultry, but go easy on red meat and dairy products such as ordinary cheese, which are much higher in fat. Get your calcium from low-fat dairy products (cottage cheese, yoghurt and skimmed milk).

- Fill up on vegetables and fruit. But be careful about fruit juice, as it is surprisingly high in sugar (and calories).

- Use an app on your phone to keep track of what you eat and drink.

So how many calories do you need?

In case you missed it earlier, an average 30-year-old woman needs around 2,000 calories a day, a bit more if she is active. By the age of 51, the average woman only needs 1,600 calories each day, though you can increase this quite a lot if you are active and do plenty of aerobic exercise.

So unless you exercise, even if you only eat 1,500 calories a day, you aren't going to lose much weight. The best way of shedding pounds once you are menopausal is to cut back to around 1,200 calories a day – so that's a 300-calorie-a-day deficit, which will mean you'll lose a pound over about 12 days. But if you add in some cardio exercise that burns 200 calories a day, every day, then on a 1,200-calorie diet you'll lose a pound in a week.

Weight, shape and body fat

I've always been careful about what I've eaten, and I've never been what any medic would call overweight, though like most women I gained a few pounds just after the menopause. I was doing a story for *BBC Breakfast* about an NHS weight-loss clinic in Rotherham and was invited to have my body fat measured. I was shocked to discover that it was 35 per cent – much higher than I had expected. I was what the doctor there called 'fat-skinny' – with a normal body weight but high body fat percentage. Worse still, like all my family, I carry any extra weight around my middle – and my waist measurement was an unhealthy 33 inches.

What had happened was I had lost muscle and gained fat, which goes to show that just standing on the scales doesn't tell the whole story about 'weight'.

It was the trigger for me to start taking more exercise, doing a mix of cardio stuff and trying to rebuild my lost muscles with weights. And now I check how I'm doing in three ways: with my body weight, my body fat percentage and also a tape measure!

Here's more detail about each of these three elements.

1) Weight and Body Mass Index
The most commonly used measure of whether you are a healthy weight is Body Mass Index, or BMI. This can give you a 'healthy weight' for your height.

A healthy BMI is between 20 and 25. A BMI of 19 is underweight, and in older women especially this increases the risk of osteoporosis. A BMI between 25 and 30 means you are overweight, and above 30 puts you in obese range.

To calculate your BMI you'll need to have your weight and height in metric measurements.

1) First take your height in metres then multiply it by itself. Write the answer down.

2) Next, weigh yourself in kilogrammes. Again, write it down.

3) Now divide your weight (step 2) by the answer from step 1. That gives your BMI.

However, as happened to me, BMI measurement alone doesn't necessarily tell the whole story. Because of the loss of muscle that occurs with increasing age, it is possible to have a BMI in the healthy range but actually to be fatter than you should be. And neither does it tell you where you are carrying your excess weight.

2) Waist measurement
It's now known that carrying excess fat around the abdominal area is a greater risk to health than having it around your hips. Women who are 'apple-shaped' have a higher risk of heart disease and diabetes

than those of the same weight and height who are 'pear-shaped', with their weight around their hips. And, of course, middle-aged spread means that nature is unkind and turns women apple-shaped in midlife.

So a simpler way to see whether you are a healthy weight is just to measure your waist, using a tape measure at the level of your tummy button. You may already know if you are an 'apple' or a 'pear' – and it's something that you can't really alter as it's something you inherit – but even if you carry most of your weight on your hips, it can still be useful to measure your waist. It should be below 32 inches. Between 32 and 35 inches means you are overweight, and above 35 inches is obese and carries with it a 30 per cent increased risk of heart disease, stroke, diabetes and arthritis.

3) Body fat

Another method that is increasingly used to check whether you are carrying too much fat is to measure what proportion of your body it makes up, using a body-fat monitor. There are various different types of machine for doing this, varying in accuracy. Unfortunately, it's only the most expensive ones, designed for professional use, that are really accurate, but even a set of scales with a body-fat monitor included can give you an idea of how your body is made up.

A healthy range of body fat for women aged 40 to 59 is 23 per cent to 34 per cent. The higher the fat percentage, the greater the risk to health. Because of the way our body changes as we get older, and because muscle is replaced by fat, it is quite possible to have a BMI in the healthy range and yet have an unhealthily high body-fat percentage – like me. If you suspect this may apply to you, body-fat scales can be especially useful. Losing weight isn't the answer, health-wise, but rather losing fat and gaining muscle.

Sophie, age 53

HER STORY: I recently tried on a 'body-con' dress and was horrified at how lumpy I looked in it. I could see flesh bulging above and below my bra, even though it felt quite comfortable, and I obviously needed control knickers to hold in my bulging tummy. I weighed myself that night and I've gained half a stone – and all of it seems to have gone around my middle. Yet nothing has really changed in my lifestyle – I go to the gym a couple of times a week and I'm quite careful with my diet. Why the change? Is it my hormones? And how much should I weigh now?

MORE BACKGROUND INFORMATION: Sophie was 5 foot 6 inches and weighed 10 stone, 11lb, so when we calculated her BMI it was 24.3, just in healthy range. But her waist measurement told a different story – even though she wore either size 12 or 14 clothes, it was 34 inches. She was horrified, she had no idea it was that large.

Her sessions at the gym involved around 20 minutes on a cross trainer, but she admitted she didn't push herself hard enough to work up much of a sweat. Then she used some of the weight machines, but because she was scared of hurting herself she kept them on low weights, which she never changed. Her diet was fairly healthy, though she didn't often eat five portions of fruit and veg each day. She also had a couple of glasses of wine a night every night, and often more at weekends.

MY ADVICE: Sophie needed to lose some of the flab that had accumulated around her middle, and in reality this meant she needed to lose at least half a stone of fat. To do this she needed first and foremost to step up her exercise regime, as what she was doing now was unfortunately not enough to either boost her metabolism or to maintain her muscles. She needed to push herself harder, and for longer, on the cross trainer, and gradually increase the weights she used on the machines. She also needed to do some work on her 'core' muscles, to tone up her tummy. I suggested she ask the gym staff for some advice – this should be free, but if she could afford it, paying for a few sessions with a personal trainer would be helpful.

Diet-wise, her top priority – for both her health and her waistline – was to cut back on the wine, to a maximum of 14 units a week, preferably less, with at least two days a week with no alcohol at all.

I suggested she monitor her progress using not only her bathroom scales, but also a tape measure. She decided she wanted to get her waist down to 30 inches, and I suggested she aim to do this over three months, no faster.

Kath, age 54

HER STORY: I've always battled with my weight, and in the past if I really try to stick to a diet I can get down between a size 12 and 14. But in the last couple of years I know the pounds have been creeping on, and now I can't get into a size 16. I've tried to cut back on my food, but it doesn't seem to make any difference. It's so depressing. My stomach is huge – I look pregnant. Why is this? Is it because of the menopause? Is there anything I can do?

MORE BACKGROUND INFORMATION: Kath was 5 foot 3 inches and weighed just over 12 stone, giving her a BMI of 30. Her waist was 38 inches. She lived in a flat and her only exercise was a short walk to the bus stop each day, plus a bit of housework once a week. She had never joined a gym because she said she couldn't afford it. She didn't eat breakfast, and tried to avoid eating anything until lunch, though sometimes she was so hungry she had a couple of biscuits. She had a sandwich and apple for lunch. She had three teenage children, who she cooked for in the evenings, and because they liked pasta or high-carbohydrate foods, she often didn't eat any herself and then found herself nibbling snacks later in the evening. When we went through her diet together, she realised she often only had one portion of either fruit or veg, and ate far too many biscuits and crisps. But on the plus side, she rarely touched alcohol.

MY ADVICE: First, she needed to start exercising. I gave her details of classes run by her council at their gym and also in the local park, but suggested that if that didn't appeal, she could try walking to or from work – the more often she could manage it, the better.

Her diet needed a lot of attention. Instead of trying to eat very little, she needed to eat more of the right type of foods, especially fruit and veg, and to make sure she had breakfast and also a proper meal on a plate in the evening, rather than just having high-fat snacks.

She needed to lose two stone and seven inches off her waist, which was a big challenge that I reckoned would sensibly take at least six months, maybe longer. I told her that slow, steady progress was far better than trying to shed too much, too fast.

Vicki, age 51

HER STORY: I've never really bothered with my weight in the past. I was a beanpole as a teenager, and though I filled out a bit after I had the kids, I've always eaten fairly sensibly, and my weight has pretty much stayed the same for the past twenty years. But in the past couple of years I've noticed my weight has been creeping up. I've gone from a size 12 to a size 14, and even though I'm being more careful what I'm eating, my new trousers and skirts are feeling tight now. I'm also feeling a bit tired, so I'm wondering if my thyroid isn't working properly. Or is it the menopause? I haven't had a period now for eight months, though I'm only having occasional flushes and sweats.

MORE BACKGROUND INFORMATION: Vicki was a tall 5 foot 10 inches and weighed just under 13 stone, giving her a BMI of 26. She had a waist of 34 inches, but was a classic apple shape, with very thin legs. Her diet was fairly well balanced, with lots of fruit and veg, and she was careful to buy semi-skimmed milk and avoid eating a lot of high-fat foods. However, she did admit she had a sweet tooth and liked puddings and chocolate. We worked out between us that on average she ate around 2,200 calories a day – sometimes a bit more, sometimes less. She worked full-time and her job involved a lot of travelling, and she also did the lion's share of the housework at home. She admitted, when asked, that she had very little time for either exercise or relaxation.

MY ADVICE: Because she was also feeling tired, it made sense to do blood tests to check for both anaemia and her thyroid function. However, both were normal so I suspected her tiredness was due to a combination of the menopause and a busy lifestyle. Her weight had crept up because she was still eating pretty much the same as she always had done, and her metabolism had fallen. Unless she took action, her weight would continue to creep upwards. To prevent further weight gain she needed to cut back to around 1,800 calories a day, and to lose weight she was going to need to cut down her calorie intake even more. She also needed to try to make some time for doing some exercise, which would boost her metabolism a bit, and allow her an occasional indulgence for her sweet tooth.

SUMMARY

It is normal for a woman's shape to change after the menopause. The lack of oestrogen means that fat tends to be laid down more around the tummy – hence that awful phrase 'middle-aged spread'.

Having a little fat around your middle is not only normal, but it's healthy, too. If you still have a 24-inch waist in your fifties, the chances are you are underweight and not only look a little gaunt but are at increased risk of osteoporosis.

Your metabolic rate falls as you get older, mainly because your muscles shrink. This means that if you eat the same at fifty as you did when you were twenty, you will put on weight. To stop yourself piling on the pounds, you need to reduce your daily calorie intake.

The best way to help control your weight is not only to watch your diet, but to take much more exercise. This should involve not only cardiovascular exercise but also doing exercises that help you maintain your muscles. Weight-bearing exercise is important, too, to help maintain strong bones.

The scales don't always tell the whole story about how healthy you are. The amount of body fat you have, and especially your waist measurement, are also important. It is possible to not be 'overweight' but still carrying too much fat for good health around your middle.

6

....

LOOKING AFTER
YOUR BONES

The menopause is often a time when women realise they are not quite in their first flush of youth any more and suddenly looking after yourself becomes more important. Though your mind may be focusing on chaotic periods and erratic moods, not to mention hot flushes and sweats that wake you every night, there is one topic that is really important – and sadly often gets forgotten – and that's your bones.

Most of us take our bones for granted and don't think about them at all, unless something happens to one of them, such as a broken arm or a creaky knee. But the reason all women should think about their bones is because of osteoporosis. It's a condition that weakens bones, making them fragile and more likely to break.

No symptoms may appear until you are in your seventies, but you really need to be aware of osteoporosis around the time of the menopause, because that is when you can best do something about it. It's a condition that affects one in three women, so it's not something you should ignore.

What I'm going to do in this chapter is explain why osteoporosis occurs, the symptoms, who is most at risk and, most importantly of all, what you can do about it.

There are lots of case histories at the end; as always, every woman is different, so hopefully these will help you to understand what you should do about your bones.

But let's start with the commonly asked questions.

What are the symptoms of osteoporosis? How will I know if I've got it?

One of the big problems with osteoporosis is that it doesn't cause any symptoms until a disaster strikes, such as a broken bone after a trivial fall. You trip on the pavement, put out your hand, and you break the arm bone just above the wrist, which would not have happened if your bones were stronger. Osteoporosis is a silent process, so there is no way you can know if you have got it. Other than a fracture, the other symptom of osteoporosis is a curved spine, which occurs because the weak bones of the spine become crushed from their normal cube shape into a wedge, causing the classic 'dowager's hump'. But this only occurs when osteoporosis is advanced.

So what about osteoarthritis, is that the same as osteoporosis?

No. Osteoarthritis is 'wear and tear' on the surfaces of bones, inside a joint. This in turn leads to pain and stiffness. It's a completely different condition from osteoporosis, and the two are not connected. You can have osteoarthritis yet have very strong bones, and conversely you can have osteoporosis and no osteoarthritis. The other really important thing to know is that osteoarthritis causes symptoms – back ache, stiff knees, aching hips. Osteoporosis is silent until a bone breaks.

Do all women get osteoporosis? Are some women more at risk than others?

One in three women get osteoporosis, so it's very common, but there are some women who aren't affected. You are more at risk of getting osteoporosis if you are of small build, or if you've gone without periods for a time because you have been underweight. You are also more at risk if there is a family history of the condition, or if you have had an early menopause (before the age of 45) and not taken HRT. Those who have coeliac disease, who have had long-term depo-contraception, taken steroid medication or had an overactive thyroid are also more at risk. But some women who have seemingly no risk factors are still affected, so all women should be aware of it.

Why is it so important at the menopause?

Yet again, it's all to do with oestrogen. Bone is living tissue, being continually broken down and rebuilt. Oestrogen helps to promote the formation of new bone, but after the menopause, this effect is lost and this means bones gradually become weaker. There is more information about this in chapter 6.

Is there a test that can show if I'm more at risk?

An ordinary X-ray may show that bones look thinner than average, but this is not a good way of diagnosing osteoporosis, and X-rays are never used for just this reason. An ultrasound of the heel bone can also indicate if the bone is thin, but the best way of checking bone density is with a DEXA (Dual Energy X-ray Absorptiometry) scan.

So how can I look after my bones?

The best way of maintaining your bones is to do regular weight-bearing exercise (see page 163) and eat a well-balanced diet that is rich in calcium. At the menopause, taking HRT can help to maintain bone strength, and bisphosphonate medication can also be used in those with confirmed severe osteopenia or osteoporosis.

Osteopenia? What is that? How is it different from osteoporosis?

Osteopenia is the medical term used to describe bones that are thinner than average, but not thin enough to be classified as osteoporosis. There is more information about this on page 158. If you have osteopenia, you are much more at risk of developing osteoporosis.

What about supplements? Should I take extra calcium?

All women need 800mg calcium each day to maintain their bones. This is best obtained from food, which also contains other micronutrients that are important for bones, such as magnesium. The best sources of calcium are dairy products, and for those worried about cholesterol, low-fat versions (such as skimmed milk) have more calcium than full fat. Fish where you eat the bones, such as sardines, are also an excellent source. You only need to take a calcium supplement if you are not getting enough in your diet. Eating mega doses of calcium is of no extra benefit, as it can't be incorporated into bones and there is some evidence that it might be harmful.

What about drugs? Is there anything I can take that will help keep my bones strong?

Yes. HRT can provide oestrogen, which can help maintain bones, and some women take it for just this reason. The other group of drugs that can help maintain bones are bisphosphonates, such as alendronic acid. There is more information about these on page 165. However, these drugs are not a cure for osteoporosis; although they may help to rebuild a little new bone, their main effect is to stop bones getting any thinner.

A BIT OF BACKGROUND ABOUT BONES

Bones are living tissues that are continually being built up by cells known as osteoblasts, and broken down by cells known as osteoclasts. In childhood, and especially the teenage years, the building-up process is more dominant. Our bones reach their maximum density in our mid-twenties, then the two processes should be fairly balanced until the thirties, when the breaking-down process becomes slightly more dominant and the bones, very gradually, become thinner. Weight-bearing exercise is important for bones throughout life for increasing bone density.

After the menopause, the loss of bone suddenly accelerates. This is because oestrogen plays a vital role in helping to maintain bone density. When oestrogen levels fall at the menopause, this protective effect is lost and bone density falls, sometimes at an alarming rate.

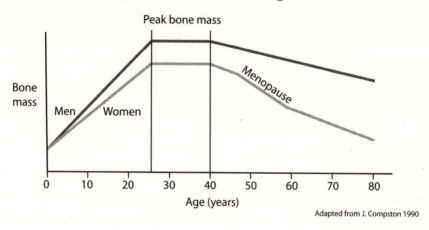

Changes in bone mass with age

Adapted from J. Compston 1990

So what do bones actually do?

I think it would be fair to say that most of us don't really take any notice of our bones – until something happens to them! We have 206 of them (plus three tiny ones in each ear) that serve as a structural frame for the body and work with ligaments, tendons and muscles to allow us to move. They also provide a protective outer shell for many internal organs, including the brain and spinal cord, as well as the heart and lungs.

Oestrogen and bones

Oestrogen has several complex actions on bone, but the most important effect is to speed the breakdown of osteoclasts, which absorb bone. When oestrogen levels fall, the osteoclasts are active for longer and this leads to increased breakdown of bone. In addition, oestrogen enhances the absorption of calcium – vital for the process of building bones – from the intestine. So at the menopause, when oestrogen levels fall, the breaking-down process becomes dominant, bone loss accelerates and bone density starts falling dramatically.

So why is osteoporosis so important?

Osteoporosis can have devastating effects on your health. Though it's rare to die of a broken bone, lying immobile in bed with a broken hip can put you at vastly increased risk of pneumonia or a deep vein thrombosis, both of which can be fatal. The statistics are horrific – every day around 40 people in the UK die as a result of an osteoporotic fracture. In addition, thousands of people – mainly women – lose their independence as a result of fractures, and crushed bones in the spine can be excruciatingly painful.

And worst of all…

Unfortunately, even with modern drugs, there is no cure for osteoporosis – once the bones are thin there is little that can be done to build them up again. Modern drugs can help stop the rot, and help prevent bones getting even thinner, but they have a very limited effect on rebuilding new bone.

So prevention is all-important, and though women of all ages should take care of their bones, you really need to be proactive about this once you reach the menopause.

WHY ME?

Sheila, age 74

'At 74, I thought I was in pretty good shape for my age. I'd kept myself fairly trim, and my love of gardening kept me active. I felt I was really lucky – so many of my friends had aching knees or backs, but I could spend hours digging the veg patch and not even have a twinge afterwards. I did notice I was getting a bit shorter, and found it a bit harder to stand up really straight, but I thought that was normal, as I'd read that the discs between the back bones got a bit thinner in later life. Then one day, out of the blue, I got the most excruciating pain in the middle of my back that went round to the front lower part of my chest. I struggled to get out of bed, took some paracetamol but it made no difference. I had to get a friend to help me to the doctor. To begin with she thought it was just wear and tear arthritis, but to be sure she arranged for me to have a back X-ray. That showed that one of vertebra at the bottom of my thoracic spine – where the ribs attach – had collapsed into a wedge shape, and that it was likely I had osteoporosis. A bone-density scan confirmed the diagnosis. I was so shocked – I had absolutely no idea anything was happening to my bones. The severe pain continued for about two months, and without really strong medication I could hardly move, but the side effects were awful – feeling tired and woozy, and bad constipation. I'm now on medication to stop my bones getting any worse, but my doctor has told me there is nothing that can be done to make my bones strong again. I've been warned to take care, as just a slight fall could mean another broken bone. Looking back at family photos I can see my grandmother and my mother couldn't stand straight when they were older, but the significance of this completely passed me by – until now. I wish I'd known about osteoporosis before. If I'd taken steps earlier, like getting a bone-density scan, and eating more calcium, it wouldn't have got this bad.'

There are lots of things that can increase the risk of osteoporosis, but they can broadly be broken down into two main groups – either not building up strong bones in the first place or having your bones break down faster, or at a younger age, than normal.

Building up strong bones in your youth is very important in helping to prevent osteoporosis, and if this didn't happen, you are more at risk in later life of developing the condition.

This can occur because of:

- Your genes. Osteoporosis can run in families, and if your mother and grandmother had it, you are likely to get it too. However, chances are members of past generations were never formally diagnosed with the condition. They just got shorter, or acquired a curved spine. So have a careful look at family photos.

- Your general build – just having a small frame, and being slim, can mean you are slightly more at risk.

- A history of anorexia, particularly during the teenage years and early twenties, and especially if your periods stopped for more than six months. This indicates that the ovaries have stopped working, and low levels of oestrogen at a time when the bones should be being built up – and aren't – can have a profound effect later in life.

- Poor nutrition and a lack of calcium – again, especially in childhood and during the teenage years when strong bones should be formed. The trend for 'no dairy' can be dangerous unless a good alternative source of calcium is incorporated into your diet.

The second group of causes, when bones start losing their strength at a younger age than normal can occur because of:

- Having an early menopause, or having your ovaries removed before the age of 45. This means an early loss of the protective effect of oestrogen, though this can be corrected by taking HRT.

- Prolonged periods of inactivity. This is because bones need exercise to maintain their density.

- Taking steroid tablets, as they have a direct effect on bone metabolism. The longer they are taken, the greater the risk of osteoporosis. However, this effect is not seen with steroid nose sprays, or with inhalers used to treat asthma, unless very high doses are used for a long period of time.

- Heavy drinking and smoking, as these can affect the way calcium is incorporated into bone.

Even though exercise is vital for both building up and maintaining strong bones, it's possible to overdo it. Excessive exercise can stop the ovaries working, with a consequent fall in oestrogen levels. If this happens in young women it can reduce the amount of bone laid down; later in life it can speed up the rate at which bone is lost. If your periods stop because of a strenuous exercise regime, your bones will suffer as a result.

What about men?

Osteoporosis doesn't just affect women – men get it too. But it's far more common in women simply because men have testosterone, which helps them build much stronger bones in their teens, and helps them to maintain them throughout their life. Bone loss is a normal part of ageing for both men and women, and by the age of 75, men and women lose bone at around the same rate. Both genders are also less able to absorb calcium. However, when men get osteoporosis, it's usually related to another health condition, or a known risk factor, such as excess smoking or drinking. In contrast, women get it simply because they never had strong bones in the first place.

DIAGNOSIS AND DEXA SCANS

The first indication that bones are thinner than they should be is often a comment on an X-ray – done for another reason, that the 'bones appear thin'. However, ordinary X-rays cannot be used to diagnose osteoporosis. A heel ultrasound can also be helpful, and is often used in private screening tests, but again it only gives an indication that the bone is thinner than it should be.

The only way to accurately diagnose osteoporosis is with a special bone-density scan. The proper name for this is 'Dual Energy X-ray Absorptiometry' – DEXA for short. This is done using a scanner which emits a very low level of radiation, and the amount that passes through your bones is then measured. The amount of radiation used is far less than a standard X-ray, and is less than two days' exposure to natural background radiation (compared to five days for a chest X-ray). It involves lying on a couch while the C-shaped scanner – one arm of the C above you, and one under the couch – passes up and down your spine and hips.

The value of a DEXA scan is that it can tell you exactly how thin your bones are, so it can be used not only to diagnose established osteoporosis, but also the earlier stages of the disease, when your bones are thinner than normal – a condition known as osteopenia.

Results

The results are usually expressed as a T score, which is a comparison with young healthy bones. There is usually a Z score as well, which is a comparison of women in the same age group (which isn't so helpful).

The scores are calculated as follows:

A T score of 1 or above is normal.

Minus 1 to minus 1.5 is a bit lower than average.

Minus 1.5 to minus 2.5 is osteopenia.

Minus 2.5 or more confirms osteoporosis.

As osteoporosis is so common, shouldn't all women have a DEXA scan?

Unfortunately there is no national screening programme for osteoporosis in the UK, and DEXA scans are only offered to those who are at increased risk of having thin bones. All women should talk through their bone health with their GP at the time of the menopause, and discuss whether they should have a DEXA scan. The other time to think about having a scan is if you break a bone after what seemed like a fairly minor fall, and certainly all women over 50 breaking their wrist or hip should have a DEXA scan done.

PREVENTION

The sooner you take action to look after your bones, the better, and osteoporosis is so horribly common that every woman should take steps to preserve her skeleton. Ideally this preparation should start in the teenage years – the stronger the bones you build in your youth, the longer they are going to last. But it's at the menopause when bone care should be part of your regular daily routine.

In simple terms, you should:

- Eat at least 800mg of calcium every day. There's more on this in the section below. That's around half a pint of milk (300ml), a pot of yoghurt and an ounce and a half of cheese.

- Make sure you are getting enough vitamin D. Again, see the separate section on page 162.

- Take regular weight-bearing exercise. There is more information about this on page 163.

- Keep your alcohol consumption under 14 units a week.

- And don't smoke.

Calcium

Calcium is a vital building block of both bones and teeth, along with a little bit of magnesium. The best source of calcium is dairy food. If you are worried about cholesterol – and your waistline – low-fat dairy such as skimmed milk, fat-free yoghurts and low-fat cheeses contain more calcium, weight for weight, than fuller-fat versions. If you are keen on dairy products, your diet may well provide you with enough. However, though green veg does contain some calcium, you have to eat mountains of them to get the significant amounts that are found in dairy products.

The only way to be sure you are getting enough calcium for your bones is to record your intake. Blood levels of calcium are carefully controlled by parathyroid hormone, and even if your intake is sub-optimal, levels in the blood are likely to be normal. They only tend to become abnormal if there is a problem with parathyroid hormone production.

Milk and dairy sources of calcium

Food	Portion size	Calcium
Whole milk	200ml	236mg
Yoghurt	125g	200mg
Cheddar cheese	30g	216mg
Soft cheese triangle	15g	100mg
Cottage cheese	100g	73mg
Skimmed milk	200ml	244mg
Ice cream	60g (one scoop)	78mg
Soy drink (non-enriched)	100ml	26mg

Non-dairy sources of calcium

Food	Portion size	Calcium
Sardines	100g (four sardines)	410mg
Pilchards	100g (two pilchards)	340mg
Haddock	150g fillet	150mg
Baked beans	220g (one half of a large can)	100mg

Food	Portion size	Calcium
Enriched soya/rice milk	200ml	240mg
Enriched orange juice	250ml	300mg
Tofu	100g	500mg
Spring green	100g	200mg
Spinach	100g	150mg
Watercress	50g	75mg
Broccoli	50g	30mg
Okra	50g	130mg
Kale	50g	65mg
Chickpeas	100g	45mg
Almonds	15g	35mg
Brazil nuts	15g	26mg
Sesame seeds	one tablespoon	160mg
Dried figs	60g (three figs)	150mg
Calcium-enriched bread	Two slices (80g)	300mg
Currants	100g	93mg

Calcium supplements

If you are not sure that you are getting 800mg of calcium a day from your food, you should take a supplement. However, there is no need to take large doses, as there is a limit to the amount of calcium that can be used to build new bone. Not only that, but high levels of calcium can impair the absorption of iron and zinc and increase the risk of developing kidney stones. High levels of calcium have been linked with an increased risk of heart disease, so it makes sense to check the labels and only take the amount you need. Calcium supplements can cause constipation and bloating, and you may need to try several different brands to find the one that you can tolerate the best.

Vitamin D

Vitamin D is required to absorb both calcium and magnesium from the gut, and also for incorporating them into bone. Only a small amount of the vitamin D we need comes from food we eat, and good sources include oily fish and eggs, and cereals that are fortified with vitamin D. However, we get most of our vitamin D from the action of sunlight on our skin.

Sunlight and vitamin D

The best way to build up your vitamin D levels is to have short daily bursts of exposure to the sun, *without sunscreen,* for 10 to 15 minutes, between 11am and 3pm. The more skin you have exposed, the more vitamin D you will make, and as long as you don't expose your skin for longer than this, you should not burn. People with darker skins need a bit longer. There is no need to expose your face without any sunscreen, though – arms and legs have a greater area of skin and aren't so prone to wrinkles!

Vitamin D is fat-soluble and can be stored in the body, so you should aim to build up your stores during the summer months, from May to September. On cloudy summer days your skin can still produce vitamin D, but it takes a little longer. Older skins are less efficient at making vitamin D, which is one of the reasons why vitamin D deficiency is very common in those over 65. You do need to make sure you are actually outside – you can't make vitamin D sitting by a window.

How can I know if I am getting enough vitamin D?

Vitamin D deficiency often does not cause any symptoms, but can lead to tiredness and muscle weakness. However, unlike calcium, a blood test for vitamin D levels can be useful in assessing whether you are getting enough. If you think you may be at risk, have your levels checked via a blood test that your GP can arrange. Vitamin D deficiency is now so common in the UK that it is recommended that everyone should have a daily supplement of 10 micrograms (400iu).

Weight-bearing exercise

This includes both cardio and strength exercises, but what is important is that your bones should be bearing your body weight, or extra weights, such as dumbbells. That means that anything in water, such as swimming, or aqua aerobics, is not included. These sports are great for toning muscles, but as the water is taking your body weight, it doesn't help your bones. Cycling isn't much good either. Weight-bearing exercises can be high or low impact. High-impact examples are hiking, jogging, tennis or doing high-impact aerobics. They are excellent for your bones, but if you already have osteoporosis, they can be risky in terms of falling and breaking a bone, in which case low-impact exercises are safer. Examples include using elliptical training machines, stair-step machines (but not exercises that involve getting on and off a step – it's too easy to miss your footing, fall over and break a bone), low-impact aerobics or fast walking, either on a treadmill or outside.

TREATMENT

Unfortunately, there is no treatment that can 'cure' osteoporosis. Once your bones are thin, there is no drug that can build them up again to any significant degree. Though in some cases it is possible to build up a little bit of new bone, the main aim of all treatment is to stop the bones getting any weaker.

Though this section is primarily about drugs, it is also important to remember that keeping your muscles strong is an important part of osteoporosis treatment. Muscles not only move your joints, but also provide a supportive role, and the stronger your muscles are, the less likely you are to have a fall that results in a broken bone.

There is more about this in the section on sarcopenia, on page 135.

HRT

The oestrogen in HRT can help preserve bones – after all, it's the loss of oestrogen at the menopause that's responsible for the fall in bone density that happens to women in their fifties. That means that HRT can be a useful treatment for women with both osteopenia and osteoporosis, especially in women in their late forties and fifties.

How long does it take?

HRT can begin to have an effect on bones straight away, but the longer it is taken, the greater its effect will be in slowing down or preventing the loss of bone that normally occurs after the menopause. Once you stop taking HRT the bones will start breaking down again at the usual higher rate that occurs in women after the menopause.

Can it be taken long term?

In terms of bones, yes, and the longer it is taken, the more prolonged the positive effect on bones. But the downside is the slightly greater risk of breast cancer and DVT, especially after five years, and even more so after 10. However, as always, it's a case of weighing up the risks – if you have thin bones a hip fracture could well pose a greater long-term danger to your health than the risk of breast cancer.

What happens to bones when you stop HRT?

HRT only works on bones while it is being taken. As soon as it is stopped, oestrogen levels fall, so bone loss starts to accelerate again.

What about side effects?

The big issue for many women taking HRT is the increased risk of breast cancer, and also, for tablets taken by mouth, the increased risk of deep vein thrombosis. Less serious but still troublesome side effects can include bloating, weight gain, breast tenderness and in some, mood changes. There is more detail about all of these in the chapter on HRT (page 59).

What about the dose? Does that matter?

Unlike treating flushes and sweats, where often a small dose of oestrogen is sufficient, to get a full benefit to your bones you will need a full-dose preparation – which is one containing 2mg oestradiol or 1.25mg conjugated oestrogens. The downside of this is the higher the dose, the greater the increased risk of breast cancer, which is why the full-dose preparations in general aren't so popular now, especially for treating flushes and sweats. However, if you have osteopenia or osteoporosis and are under 60, taking HRT can be a good way of stopping your bones getting worse. And of course it can have other benefits, too, such as stopping flushes and sweats and maintaining libido. However, as with those who take it for other symptoms, any woman taking HRT needs to be warned that flushes and sweats can be a problem when they stop taking it, and this should be done very gradually, especially with the higher-dose preparations used to protect bones.

Bisphosphonates

These are the most popular drugs used for treating severe osteopenia and osteoporosis.

There are several different bisphosphonates available, but the most popular are alendronic acid and risedronic acid, which are taken weekly, and ibandronic acid, which is taken once a month. Zoledronic acid is an intravenous preparation which is only used for those with severe osteoporosis, where other treatments are not suitable. It is given once a year.

How do they work?

They work by slowing down the action of osteoclasts, the cells that break down bone. This allows the osteoblasts (the ones that build bone) to work more effectively. There is good evidence that taking bisphosphonates can help to prevent bone becoming weaker, and in some they can also build up a little new bone.

How long does it take?

It takes several months for bisphosphonates to work, but there usually is a slight increase in bone density between six and 12 months after you start taking them, and bone density can improve by 2 to 3 per cent over a two-year period.

Can they be taken long term?

No. Exactly how long bisphosphonates should be taken for is a subject of much debate, as research has suggested that prolonged use can alter the bone-making process and may lead to development of weak bone that is more prone to fractures. To get the best bone-building effect, most doctors suggest that they are taken for at least five years, but after this your bones should be reassessed. For some with severe osteoporosis it may be worth continuing longer than this, but they certainly shouldn't be taken for years and years on end without regular assessment.

So what happens when you stop taking them?

Bisphosphonates continue working on bones for a few years after the medicine has been stopped, so there is no need to be alarmed if your doctor suggests you should stop taking them – as long as you continue to exercise and eat enough calcium your bones should not get worse.

What about side effects?

The main side effects of bisphosphonates are that they can cause inflammation of the lower end of the oesophagus, which leads to a pain similar to severe indigestion behind the breastbone. They also have been linked with a problem with the jaw bone – osteonecrosis of the jaw. In this, the blood supply to the jawbone is reduced, and the bones cells die. It tends to occur after a tooth is removed. It is an incredibly rare condition, but there does seem to be an increased risk in those who have had high-dose bisphosphonates. The main people affected are those who have had bisphosphonates intravenously, usually as part of treatment for cancer.

Because of this, any woman who is recommended bisphosphonates should always have a dental check-up and any necessary dental work done before starting treatment. Make sure you tell your dentist if you are already on bisphosphonates if you need to have invasive dental work done, such as an implant or tooth removal.

How are they taken?

Bisphosphonates aren't absorbed when taken with food, they have to be taken on an empty stomach with a glass of water, and to avoid problems with the oesophagus, you must take them sitting upright, then stay upright for the next hour. There's no waking early in the morning, taking your pill then going back to bed for an hour, or taking them with an early cup of tea an hour before breakfast. The good news is that they only need to be taken either once a week or once a month, so you don't have this palaver every day.

OTHER DRUGS

The main drugs used for osteopenia and osteoporosis are bisphosphonates and HRT, but there are some others that are occasionally used.

Raloxifene is a selective oestrogen receptor modulator (SERM for short). To translate that into plain English, it means it stimulates the oestrogen receptors in bone, but blocks the oestrogen receptors on other organs, such as the womb and, most importantly, the breasts. Though this sounds great in theory, in practice it's not as effective as bisphosphonates, and weirdly seems to have a better effect on the bones of the spine than the hips. In the UK it is only licensed for use to reduce the risk of spinal fracture if bisphosphonates are not suitable. It's taken as a daily tablet. Hot flushes can be a troublesome side effect.

Denosumab is one of a group of drugs known as 'monoclonal human antibodies', biological therapies that are made in laboratories and which target specific proteins on the outside of cells. Denosumab blocks a protein called RANKL which controls the activity of osteoclasts, the cells that break down bone. The effect is to stop bone being broken down. It's given by injection twice a year. Like bisphosphonates, Denosumab can increase very slightly the risk of osteonecrosis of the jaw, and can also increase the risk of general infections and cause rashes and sweating. It's only used in those with established osteoporosis in whom bisphosphonates are unsuitable.

Parathyroid hormone (PTH) is produced naturally by the body to help in the regulation of levels of calcium in the body, which also stimulates osteoblasts (which form new bone). It's an expensive treatment that can be given to those with severe osteoporosis in whom other treatments are unsuitable. It's given by injection, and only by hospital specialists, and blood calcium levels have to be carefully monitored afterwards.

Strontium appears to have an action on both osteoblasts and osteoclasts, and can help stop loss of bone. However, it can increase the risk of heart attacks, and for this reason it is rarely used.

Getting treatment

The official guidance about who should be given treatment is complicated and depends on several factors. Certainly anyone with confirmed osteoporosis on a DEXA scan should be offered treatment, but treatment should also be given to those with osteopenia who have additional risk factors, such as taking oral steroids or a previous fracture. As with so many medical conditions, different doctors interpret the guidelines differently, and some GPs are much more willing to prescribe treatment than others. It helps to see a GP who has a special interest in the menopause and osteoporosis. If you want to get more information, look at the chart published by the National Osteoporosis Guideline Group (NOGG).

FRACTURE PREVENTION

Any discussion about osteoporosis would not be complete without mentioning fracture prevention. If you know you have osteopenia or osteoporosis, it makes sense to take steps to reduce your risk of breaking a bone.

If you've had a DEXA scan and been told your T score is in the minus range, it's probably the time to reassess whether you want to continue activities that put you at increased risk of ending up with a plaster on your arm, such as horse riding or skiing. You may decide that you prefer to carry on enjoying yourself and take the risk, but it's worth having a think about it.

But more important is to strengthen your muscles, which are essential for strength and balance.

So that is all the theory. But how is it put into practice?

Here are some case histories that will hopefully help you to make sense of it all.

Janey, age 51

HER STORY: My periods stopped a few months ago, and I'm having terrible flushes and sweats. I'm also a bit worried about my bones. I had mild anorexia when I was younger and my periods stopped for about a year when I was doing my A levels. I eat properly now, but I like to keep myself trim. I wonder if I should be checked for osteoporosis?

MORE BACKGROUND INFORMATION: Janey was indeed very trim, she only weighed 8 stone, and at a height of 5 foot 2 inches that gave her a Body Mass Index of 20 – right at the lower end of the normal range. She said that if anything she was 'fatter than normal', so she had clearly always been slightly underweight, and she admitted she avoided dairy foods as she regarded them as fattening. She went to the gym twice a week and did a mix of cardio and weight exercises. She also enjoyed playing tennis.

MY ADVICE: Janey's lack of periods when she was younger meant she had no oestrogen for a year in her late teens, a time when she should have been building up her bones, and this, together with her very trim figure and small frame, meant that she was at risk of having thinner bones than average.

I arranged for her to have a DEXA scan, which showed she had osteopenia; her spine and both her hips had a density well below normal, though not quite bad enough to be classified as osteoporosis.

I explained that as her periods had now stopped, her bone density would start to decline faster and she would soon become osteoporotic.

The best option for Janey was to start HRT. This would help to stop her bones becoming any thinner, and would also help stop her flushes and sweats. Though in general the lowest dose is used for treating menopausal symptoms, for protecting bones it's better to have a full dose.

The higher the dose, the greater the risk of breast cancer, and this risk would also be increased by progesterone. So I suggested we keep the dose of progesterone going to her breasts as low as possible by fitting a Mirena coil. This would keep the womb lining thin, but would minimise the amount of progesterone going to her breasts. She decided she preferred taking the oestrogen by mouth, so I prescribed her 2mg daily of estradiol. I suggested that in order to minimise side effects she should start by cutting them in half for the first month, to give her body a chance to adapt to the sudden increase in oestrogen.

In the longer term, I suggested that she stay on HRT for five years, maybe longer, with repeat bone scans every three years. As long as she took plenty of weight-bearing exercise and had plenty of calcium, her bones should stay stable while she was on HRT. When she stopped the HRT her bone density would fall, and then she could consider taking a bisphosphonate instead.

Mandy, age 54

HER STORY: My older sister has just been diagnosed with osteoporosis and been put on weekly tablets. She told me it could run in families, so I thought I should come and see you, especially as my right knee has been hurting a bit recently when I've been on my feet all day. But other than that I feel fine, and in honesty, I've never even thought about my bones until she called me.

MORE BACKGROUND INFORMATION: Mandy was slim, but had never been underweight, and her periods had been regular until they stopped when she was 50. She did regular Pilates but no other exercise, and avoided eating dairy food as a way of trying to avoid putting on weight, which meant she was actually eating very little calcium on a day-to-day basis.

MY ADVICE: Because of her family history, I arranged for her to have a DEXA scan, which showed that her bone density was slightly below normal for her age and just into the range of osteopenia.

She was not having any menopausal symptoms, and between us we decided that on the basis of her bones alone she did not really need to take HRT. Nor were her bones bad enough for her to need bisphosphonates. What she did need to do, though, was make lifestyle changes to try to maintain her bones as much as possible. That meant doing some regular weight-bearing exercise and increasing her calcium intake to at least 800mg a day. I emphasised that low-fat dairy foods, such as skimmed milk and cottage cheese, were low in calories and high in calcium, but to be on the safe side she decided to take a calcium supplement as well as making changes to her diet. We agreed to monitor her bones by repeating her DEXA scans every three years, and if her bone density fell significantly, she should consider starting a bisphosphonate.

Sandra, age 61

HER STORY: I broke my wrist last week. All I did was trip over my phone cable and landed slightly awkwardly on my arm. It was such a silly little fall, but now I'm in plaster for six weeks. The specialist suggested I should come and discuss with you whether my bones have become weak.

MORE BACKGROUND INFORMATION: Up until her fall Sandra had been fit and well. She was slightly plump, ate well, but she admitted she had put on weight in her fifties and used to be quite thin. She couldn't remember exactly when her periods had started, but knew it was later than most of her friends at school, and they had stopped when she was 45. This hadn't really bothered her at the time, as she had very little in the way of flushes and sweats and her family was complete. When I asked about her family, she admitted that her mother, who had died at least 15 years ago, had developed very rounded shoulders and become a lot shorter, but again she had not attached any significance to this.

MY ADVICE: The fact that Sandra had broken a bone after a trivial fall suggested she might have osteoporosis, and this was confirmed by a DEXA scan, which showed her T score was minus 2.7 in both her spine and her hips. I checked her calcium and vitamin D levels, and these were both normal. She understandably wanted to know why her bones had become so thin, and I explained it was impossible to be exactly sure, but she had only had the beneficial effect of oestrogen on her bones for 30 years – about 10 years less than average. Added to this she had been quite thin, which may have played a part, together with her genes – it sounded as if her mother probably had osteoporosis in her spine.

Having confirmed osteoporosis, and having had a fracture, it was essential that Sandra had treatment to stop her bones getting any worse. I advised that she should take alendronic acid, once a week, but have a dental check and have any treatment she needed done before she started the tablets. In addition, I suggested it was important she maintained her calcium and vitamin D levels, and to be sure that she was getting enough I prescribed her a calcium and vitamin D supplement. She also needed to do regular weight-bearing exercise, but because her bones were fragile, I advised she avoided sports where she was at risk of another fall and fracture, such as walking or jogging on slippery surfaces, or doing step-aerobic classes (where it is all too easy to miss the step!). I advised that she should have another DEXA scan in three years' time to check that her bones were not getting any worse.

SUMMARY

☐ Osteoporosis is very common, affecting one in three women at some stage in their life.

☐ It does not cause any symptoms at all until it is at an advanced stage. Unlike osteoarthritis, it does not cause joint pain, and there is no way of knowing you have it in the early stages.

☐ The most common way by which women discover they have osteoporosis is when they break a bone after a trivial fall. Osteoporosis can also cause a curved spine and loss of height, but only when the bones are already very weak.

☐ Oestrogen helps to maintain bones, so bones suddenly start becoming weaker after the menopause.

☐ There is no cure for osteoporosis – once bones have become thin there is no treatment that can build them back up again, the available treatments just aim to stop further bone loss.

☐ Some women are more at risk than others of having osteoporosis. This includes those with a small build, or who have had an early menopause, or whose periods stopped because of low weight or excessive exercise, or who have a family history of the condition.

☐ Prevention is all-important, and that means eating at least 800mg of calcium a day, making sure your vitamin D levels are adequate and doing regular weight-bearing exercise.

7

....

MENSTRUAL MAYHEM

The first sign that the menopause is approaching is usually a change in the pattern of periods. Some women just find their periods become lighter, and more spaced apart, but others find they just stop, out of the blue. More commonly, though, what was once a regular predictable menstrual bleed may become completely erratic, with bleeding of variable heaviness seemingly occurring at random, and sudden, really heavy bleeds, soaking through everything you are wearing, may also make a very unwelcome appearance. For some women, the menstrual mayhem that occurs around the time of the change can be really distressing. The good news is that it doesn't go on forever and there are things you can do about it.

So, as before, I'll start with the questions I'm often asked in my surgery, then go on to the background biology about hormones and also specific conditions that can affect periods, such as fibroids and endometriosis. And in each section there is information about the treatments available as well as a few case histories with personal experiences of this change.

The commonly asked questions:

My periods are all over the place, which has never happened before. I never know when I'm going to start bleeding. How long is this going to carry on?

Unfortunately there is no quick and easy answer to this. This sort of pattern usually starts when the ovaries are no longer functioning properly, in the run-up to the menopause. In some women it only lasts a few months, in others about a year. It is unusual for menopausal-related menstrual havoc to last much longer than this, though occasionally it can.

I missed a period and then had one that was so heavy I couldn't leave the house. Why has this happened? Is it likely to happen again?

This usually happens because the ovaries are not functioning properly and ovulation has not occurred. This means that the ovaries have not produced any progesterone. Some oestrogen is still being produced, though, and this stimulates continuous build-up of the lining of the womb. Eventually this thickened lining becomes unstable and breaks down, causing a horrendously heavy period. There is more information about this on page 179.

I went for five months without a period, and thought they had finished, then suddenly had another one. When are they finally going to stop?

Probably pretty soon, assuming your cycle was fairly regular before. A long gap of five months suggests your ovaries really are winding down and you may not have another period. But don't throw away your sanitary towels just yet, as it's possible you may have another bleed in a couple of months.

My periods have always been a bit erratic, but now it seems to be a bit worse. I'll have two in a month, then a gap of a couple of months. Is this the menopause?

If you have always had an erratic cycle it can be really difficult to know when you are becoming perimenopausal. A blood test for your FSH level can sometimes be helpful, but it needs to be done during a period, which can be difficult if you never know when you are going to have one! If your FSH is above 15, it would suggest you are perimenopausal.

I'm in my mid-forties and in the last few years my periods have got heavier and heavier. I often have to wear a tampon and a pad, and I often pass clots. Is this dangerous? What's causing this? Is it the menopause?

Heavy periods, month after month, are not usually caused by the menopause. Especially at your age, something else is likely to be to blame, such as fibroids, or adenomyosis. There is more information about these on page 182. The main risk from this type of bleeding is that it can cause iron-deficiency anaemia, which is common in women in their forties. This type of bleeding needs to be checked out by your doctor.

I keep spotting in between periods and after sex. It's been going on for several months now. Is this normal for the menopause?

No. Though erratic bleeding is common around the time of the menopause, it should take the form of definite bleeds, varying from a light to a heavy period. Spotting – just odd bits of blood – is not normal, particularly if it's happening on a repeated basis. This type of bleeding should always be checked out by a doctor, as it can be a sign of an infection, a polyp in the womb, or something more serious, such as cancer.

SO WHAT ON EARTH IS GOING ON?

As fewer follicles remain in the ovaries and they become less responsive to FSH, it can take longer for an egg to ripen. It may take three or four weeks, or maybe even as long as three months, resulting in a much longer gap between periods. Sometimes the egg is released at the normal time, but the post-ovulatory (luteal) phase shortens and a period occurs slightly earlier than before.

Alternatively, no egg is released at all – an 'anovulatory cycle'. When this happens, the ovaries continue to produce oestrogen, which stimulates the growth of the womb lining, but there is no balancing effect from progesterone. Instead, the womb lining just keeps on getting thicker until it becomes unstable and breaks down. The timing of this is completely haphazard – sometimes two weeks after the last period, sometimes much longer. Because the ovaries wind down in a very erratic fashion, there may be a few weeks when they are producing very little oestrogen. Then they wake up a bit, and oestrogen production starts up again. So it's possible to have an anovulatory cycle after three months or even longer. The result, though, is usually an extremely heavy period, at a completely unpredictable time, often with large clots. It's why all women of a certain age should carry sanitary protection with them at all times! It's only when you've had a gap of six months of more from a period that you are likely to have stopped for good.

Are erratic periods dangerous?

Erratic periods can be a real nuisance, but they aren't dangerous. 'Toxins' don't build up in the womb lining, and there is actually no biological need to have a period once a month. Having periods less frequently can actually be a good thing, as you are less likely to become deficient in iron, but of course the opposite is true if you have months on end of periods every two to three weeks, especially if the bleeding is heavy.

And it's not always the menopause ...

Erratic periods can occur for other reasons and if you are in your early forties it's especially important not to assume that the menopause is to blame. They can occur in polycystic ovary syndrome (PCOS) and also be linked to either an overactive or especially an underactive thyroid. The ovaries also may not function normally in women who are either underweight or overweight, and in women who take a lot of exercise. Severe stress can also send your hormone cycle out of kilter, though this is not nearly as common as it is sometimes made out to be.

Erratic periods can also occur in women using progesterone-based contraceptive methods, particularly the progesterone-only pill and the implant, as these can interfere with ovulation.

Be wary of bleeding in between periods

Odd spotting between periods – a couple of days here, a couple of days there – can occasionally occur in the run-up to the menopause. But it shouldn't be happening repeatedly. Bleeding between periods is often a sign that a polyp has developed from the womb lining. This is a fleshy growth, a bit like a grape. Polyps usually aren't cancerous, but they do need to be removed and examined to be absolutely sure. So don't assume that bleeding in between periods is due to the menopause. Go to your doctor and get it checked out – which usually means having an ultrasound scan.

HEAVY PERIODS

In the next section I'm going to give more information about the commonest problem of all for women in their forties – heavy periods.

I'll explain what causes them and also, very importantly, what you can do about them.

Isobel, age 55

'I'd been feeling tired for ages – just cleaning the house made me exhausted. My periods had got a bit heavier, too, and on the first day or two of each period I had to wear a pad as well as a tampon, but I thought that was normal for my age. I was 47, and thought I might be approaching the menopause. But when I fell asleep during book club one evening my girlfriends told me, quite firmly, that I needed to see my GP. I didn't mention my periods to him to begin with – it wasn't exactly the sort of thing I wanted to discuss with a middle-aged bloke. He arranged some blood tests and it showed I was really anaemic, and my iron levels were really low. He then asked about my bleeding, and when I told him what had been happening, he wanted to do an internal examination. I couldn't face that, so we agreed he could prod my tummy. He said my womb felt enlarged and arranged for me to have a scan. Thankfully it was a woman doing it – I know it's silly but even after having three kids I'm still not happy about revealing my private bits to men. She told me I had several fibroids which were altering the shape of the lining of my womb, which was why my periods were so heavy.

I then had to decide what to do about it. My doctor suggested I see a gynaecologist, but I really didn't want any surgery, and I reckoned if I could sort out my anaemia and tiredness, I could cope. I never wear trousers on the first couple of days of my period, and always have a good supply of tampons and towels at home and work and keep some spares in my handbag as well. My doctor has given me norethisterone hormone tablets which I take to delay my period if I'm going on holiday, which is really helpful. So that's what I'm doing at the moment. I'm on iron supplements, and I know that while I'm still having heavy periods I need to continue with them, but I reckon I can manage this for another three years. I know it's not what most women want, but for me the menopause will be a relief – I just hope it comes early, and not when I'm in my mid-fifties!'

How do I know if my periods are heavy? I don't know what's normal for other women!

It can be difficult to know if you are really having heavy periods – after all, no woman goes around looking at other women's sanitary towels. And what seems heavy for one woman may be normal for another.

Studies have been done on menstrual flow – brave women have given their used sanitary pads to researchers who have carefully weighed them and worked out how much blood they contain. A 'normal' period is between 20 and 60ml (4 to 12 teaspoonfuls), while a heavy period is classified as being 60ml or more.

However, there are easier, admittedly less scientific, ways of judging whether your periods are heavy or not. If you soak through a super tampon or towel in two hours, if you need to wear two pads at once or if you pass several clots larger than a grape, the flow is heavier than average. Most women have a day or two of heavy flow during their periods, especially in the run-up to the menopause, but it's not normal to have heavy flow for four or more days. Similarly, periods on average last five days. If yours are going on for more than a week, chances are you are shedding more blood than average.

Are they dangerous?

Heavy periods can just seem like a nuisance, especially if you want to wear light clothing. But apart from the cost of all that sanitary protection, repeated heavy periods can drain your iron stores very fast and are a common cause of anaemia. They can also be a sign of an underlying gynaecological problem.

So why are they happening?

The most common reason for an occasional heavy period in the run-up to the menopause is an anovulatory cycle. But the key to anovulatory cycles is that they are erratic and often interspersed with more normal periods. Anovulation cannot be blamed for heavy periods that are regular.

The womb does tend to get slightly larger with increasing age, particularly after having a baby, and women often notice their periods get a little heavier in their thirties and forties.

Heavy periods can be a sign of a pelvic infection, but that nearly always causes other telltale symptoms as well, such as more painful periods and pelvic pain, particularly during and after sex. Polyps can also cause slightly heavier periods than normal, though they rarely cause really heavy periods with clots. However, in many women there is no clearly identifiable cause for heavy periods, especially in the years in the approach to the menopause. Gynaecologists call it 'dysfunctional uterine bleeding', and it's almost certainly due to changes in the balance between the levels of oestrogen and progesterone.

What about fibroids?

One of the most common causes of heavy periods in women in their forties and early fifties is fibroids.

These are balls of muscle and fibrous tissue that develop in the wall of the womb. They are usually quite small, often only the size of a pea, but they can grow very large, to the size of a grapefruit. There may be just one, or several.

Fibroids are common – at least 20 per cent of women over 30 have at least one, but many are unaware they have them. They are much more common in Afro-Caribbean women, in whom they have a tendency to grow to a large size. No one knows why some women get them and others don't, but they do grow in response to oestrogen and progesterone. This means that they often develop during pregnancy, when hormone levels are high, but they shrink after the menopause, when hormone levels fall.

Fibroids are not dangerous – they never turn cancerous – but they can cause discomfort in the lower abdomen, especially if they are large and if so they can cause a noticeable bulge, similar in appearance to the early stages of pregnancy. Large fibroids can also press on the bladder, making you feel you need to pee more frequently. Fibroids can cause heavy periods, especially if they distort the womb lining, and make periods more painful. But they should not affect your cycle, which is how often you have periods, as they don't alter hormone levels.

And endometriosis and adenomyosis?

In endometriosis, tissue similar to the womb lining is found elsewhere in the body. The most common places are in the pelvis, on the ligaments that support the womb, around the fallopian tubes and in and around the ovaries. Endometriotic tissue can also occur within the wall of the womb, a condition called adenomyosis. More rarely, endometriosis occurs in the bowel, the bladder or even in the tummy button.

Endometriotic tissue responds to the monthly changes in hormone levels, just like the womb lining, and thickens then bleeds at the time of a period. Any blood that is shed inside the pelvis is trapped, and though only tiny amounts are shed, it irritates the surrounding tissues, causing inflammation and pain. The same happens if bleeding occurs in the wall of the womb.

The most common symptoms of endometriosis and adenomyosis is pain, which classically builds up for a few days before each period, and is at its worst during the first day or two of bleeding. The pain can be really severe, and difficult to control, even with strong painkillers. Some women experience pain or a dull ache in the pelvis at other times, and find deep penetration during intercourse very uncomfortable. Other symptoms can include low back pain and also pain passing urine. Interestingly, though, endometriosis doesn't always cause symptoms – some women are found to have it quite by chance when they have pelvic surgery for an unrelated reason. Not only that, but the amount of endometriosis that a woman has doesn't always correlate with her symptoms – some women have dreadful pain, but when they have surgery are found only to have a few tiny spots of endometriotic tissue, while others have large areas of tissue with hardly any symptoms at all.

Endometriosis and infertility

Endometriosis is linked with infertility, but the exact association is unclear, unless the fallopian tubes are scarred. Plenty of women who have the condition are able to conceive without difficulty and one study showed that 22 per cent of women being sterilised after completing their families were found to have endometriotic deposits.

The exact cause of endometriosis is also unclear, but the most popular theory is that it is due, in some way, to 'retrograde menstruation'. During a period, some blood flows backwards up through the fallopian tubes and spills into the pelvic cavity, but in most women this is mopped up by white blood cells from the immune system. A combination of a deficit in the cleaning-up process, plus slight differences in hormone levels, means the deposits remain in some women.

Though endometriosis often causes symptoms in younger women, adenomyosis may only rear its head in the perimenopause, causing heavy, painful periods.

Can heavy periods be due to cancer?

It would be wrong to write about heavy periods and not mention cancer, but it's incredibly rare for cancer of the womb to just cause heavy periods. There are nearly always other symptoms as well, usually bleeding in between periods or a bloody discharge. Similarly, cancer of the other pelvic organs – the cervix, the ovaries or the fallopian tubes – does not present with heavy periods.

Do I need any tests?

Blood tests that can be useful include checking FSH and LH levels, to get some sort of idea if you are menopausal, but as levels can vary so much these are best done during a period. Blood tests should also be done to check levels of thyroid hormone and your iron levels.

All women with heavy periods should have a basic pelvic examination done by their GP, though to be honest some GPs are way more experienced in this than others. In some practices, you will be referred to the in-house doctor known to have the best gynaecological skills. The examination should include a check of the appearance of the cervix, using a speculum. This is a tubular device with two rounded sides that can be prised apart and which is passed into the vagina, then gently opened. The doctor will be looking for polyps at the entrance to the cervical canal, or any other abnormalities. It's a good time to have a cervical smear if you are due one but smears are not done as part of a check for abnormal bleeding.

The doctor should then do a 'bimanual examination', which, as its name implies, involves both the examiner's hands. The first and second fingers of the right hand are placed in the vagina, the fingers of the left hand are placed on the lower abdomen, and the womb and ovaries can be felt between them. It's usually possible to detect if the womb is enlarged, or if there are fibroids, though this can be difficult in women who are overweight.

The next step is a pelvic ultrasound scan. This can give a detailed image of the pelvic organs and can be particularly useful for identifying any abnormalities in the womb, such as thickening of the lining, fibroids or adenomyosis.

And what can be done about heavy periods?

This depends on the underlying cause, but here are some of the options.

When considering what to do, it's very important to consider your age and when your periods are likely to stop naturally of their own accord. An FSH measurement may be helpful with this, though as I've said previously, it can vary enormously from day to day, so if the result is borderline, it may be worth having it done more than once.

What you really want to know is how long your heavy periods are likely to carry on. If it's unlikely to be more than a year, it's probably worth trying to stick with medical methods, even if they don't seem to be particularly effective. But if you are in your mid-forties and your FSH level is normal, you could well be faced with another five years of period trouble – and that's a different ball game altogether. Your GP or gynaecologist can hopefully give you some guidance on this – inevitably judging when the menopause is going to happen is easier in some cases than others.

Medical options for treatment

- **Non-steroidal anti-inflammatory drugs** (NSAIs) can help reduce bleeding a little. They work by reducing the production of prostaglandin chemicals within the womb. For best effect they should be started two days before a period is due, but if you are perimenopausal and your cycle has become erratic, that's easier said than done. Don't wait until the bleeding becomes heavy – just start them as soon as you begin to bleed and continue while heavy bleeding persists. Traditionally the one prescribed by doctors has been mefenamic acid, but that's mainly because the drug company that made the original trade version (Ponstan) did trials on both period pains and bleeding. It's probable that other NSAIs, such as ibuprofen, work just as well, and unlike mefenamic acid, it can be bought directly from chemists.

- **Tranexamic acid** can also be helpful. Despite the rather confusing similarity in name to mefenamic acid, this is a completely different drug. It works by closing down the tiny blood vessels in the womb lining that bleed during menstruation. It only needs to be taken during the duration of heavy bleeding and is available both on prescription and from chemists. It can be taken together with NSAIs for additional effect.

- Taking the **combined contraceptive pill** (often referred to as the COCP) can dramatically reduce menstrual blood flow and can also help to regulate an erratic cycle. It can be taken right up until the menopause but is not suitable for all women. See page 210 for more details.

- **The Mirena Intrauterine System** (IUS) is increasingly used to control heavy periods in perimenopausal women. It works by thinning the womb lining and can have a dramatic effect on reducing menstrual blood losses. However, in the first few months after insertion it can cause frequent, sometimes almost continuous, bleeding, though this should not be heavy.

- Frequent heavy bleeding caused by anovulatory cycles can sometimes be helped by taking a **synthetic progesterone** for two weeks each month. This helps to counteract the 'oestrogen-only' effect and can help to regulate periods, as bleeding should only occur at the end of each course of progesterone. So it's possible to regulate the cycle to one period a month, but unfortunately this doesn't usually make much overall difference to blood flow – periods can still be just as heavy.

What about HRT for period problems?

HRT contains low doses of hormones which are not enough to override the hormones being produced by the ovaries. This is in contrast to the combined pill, which contains much higher doses of hormones, enough to stop the ovaries working. If you are still having periods when you start HRT, you will need to take a 'cyclical regime' of oestrogen, then have progesterone added in for at least 10 days each month. This produces a bleed at the end of each course of progesterone, but this won't necessarily make periods any lighter, or improve unpredictable periods. That means that HRT should not be used primarily as a treatment for heavy or erratic periods.

That doesn't mean HRT can't be used if your periods are trouble-some and you are getting hot flushes or sweats, but it is always important to rule out other causes of heavy periods before starting HRT. There is more information about this in a case history on page 89.

Surgical options

Unless there is an obvious reason for heavy periods that won't be sorted out by medical treatments – for example, large fibroids that are distorting the womb lining – surgery is usually only considered if medical options have failed.

In the past, a dilatation and curettage (usually shorted to D and C), which scraped away the womb lining, was often performed. However, this is now obsolete, simply because it didn't work for more than a month or two – the womb lining just grew back.

The new version of the D and C is a hysteroscopy, where a tiny camera is passed inside the womb under an anaesthetic, allowing the gynaecologist to view the womb cavity and lining. It is mainly done as an aid to diagnosis because a sample can also be taken of the womb lining, but it can be used for treatment, for removing polyps that are causing heavy bleeding.

Removing the womb lining

In cases where there is no obvious cause for heavy periods, one possible treatment is to burn away most of the womb lining. There are several ways of doing this. The first method developed uses a heated electrical wire which is passed into the uterus via a hysteroscope. Known as transcervical resection of the endometrium (TCRE), it's performed under a general anaesthetic on a day-case basis. In up to 40 per cent of women, periods stop altogether after the procedure, and in most of the others, blood flow during periods is markedly reduced. However, up to 5 per cent of women undergoing the procedure continue to have heavy periods, in which case the options are to either have a repeat procedure or have a hysterectomy.

More recently, a popular way of destroying the endometrium involves inserting a balloon into the womb cavity, then filling it with hot water. Other techniques include freezing the lining, or heating it with a microwave probe. However, these techniques are not as effective as TCRE and cannot be used in women with fibroids that protrude into the womb cavity.

Treating fibroids

The treatment for fibroids depends very much on their size and position. Small and medium-sized fibroids that are causing minimal distortion to the lining of the womb can be left alone, especially in perimenopausal women, as they will shrink naturally once oestrogen levels fall after the menopause.

Small fibroids that are causing heavy periods because they are distorting the womb lining can often be removed via a hysteroscopy – transcervical resection. Women having this done need to discuss their individual risk carefully with their gynaecologist – the larger the fibroid, the greater the chance of heavy bleeding both during and after the procedure.

In women who have large fibroids and who are keen to maintain their fertility, removing them may be an option – a myomectomy procedure. However, again, the larger the fibroid, the greater the risk of bleeding. It's not an operation that is usually done in women in their perimenopausal years, whose natural fertility is very low. Having a hysterectomy is far safer.

For large, troublesome fibroids, hysterectomy is usually the best treatment, though to make the operation easier it's normal to shrink the fibroids first. This makes them technically much easier to remove.

Fibroids can be shrunk using drugs that stop production of oestrogen and progesterone. The most common method is to use GnRH analogues (Gonadotropin-releasing hormone analogues). These switch off the ovaries, causing a dramatic fall in oestrogen. This does, though, usually cause menopausal side effects, particularly flushes and sweats. With fibroids, the treatment is usually given as a monthly injection.

The second drug used for shrinking fibroids is ulipristal acetate. This blocks the action of progesterone, but this alone seems to be effective in many women in shrinking fibroid size.

The problem for many women is the drugs can't be used long term. GnRH analogues can only be given for three months because it usually causes severe side effects, particularly flushes and sweats. Ulipristal is also only given for three months at a time, though it is possible to give up to four intermittent courses. Once either drug has been stopped, the fibroids have a habit of regrowing.

Research has shown that after a three-month course of treatment many women get symptom relief for up to six months afterwards. So if you are nearing the menopause it may be possible to use either GnRH analogues or, better still, ulipristal as an interim measure, in the hope that nature intervenes, natural hormone production stops and the fibroids slowly then shrink of their own accord. That said, fibroids shrink quite slowly after the menopause, so if they are large enough to make your abdomen feel uncomfortable, or they are pressing on your bladder and making you pee more often, these symptoms may continue for years after your periods stop.

Another way of treating fibroids is to cut off their blood supply, a method known as uterine artery embolisation. This involves passing a thin flexible tube under X-ray guidance into the artery that supplies the fibroid via the large artery in the leg. A chemical is then injected that blocks the artery. Following this the fibroid gradually shrinks, and though this can take six to nine months, many women notice an improvement in their symptoms within three months. There is a small risk of infection occurring after the procedure, which may require treatment with intravenous antibiotics.

Newer techniques to treat fibroids are constantly being developed. MRI-guided focused ultrasound uses pulses of high-power ultrasound waves. There is evidence this can work in the short term, but long-term results are not yet known. MRI-guided laser ablation is similar, using laser energy passed down a small needle to destroy the fibroid. Again, long-term results are not known.

Treating adenomyosis and endometriosis

The aim of treatment here is to starve the endometriotic and adeno-myotic tissue of the cycle of hormones that stimulate their growth. Taking the combined contraceptive pill can be helpful, especially if several months of treatment are taken continuously, without a break. Though this contains both oestrogen and progesterone, the effects of the two balance each other out and growth of endometriotic tissue slows down. Better still, especially for adenomyosis, is the Mirena IUS, which releases progesterone into the womb and shrinks both the womb lining and the endometriotic tissue inside the womb muscle. Progesterone-only contraceptive pills, which are taken continuously, can also be helpful, but erratic bleeding can be a troublesome side effect.

GnRH analogues are drugs which block the production of FSH and LH from the pituitary and so 'switch off' the ovaries. They are given either by nasal spray or by injection, usually for six months. They can induce sudden menopausal symptoms due to the fall in oestrogen levels, but these can be alleviated by giving a small quantity of continuous oestrogen and progesterone (in the form of low-dose HRT). This 'add-back' treatment does not appear to reduce the effectiveness of the treatment.

Unfortunately, it is rare for any medical treatment to get rid of endometriotic tissue completely – it merely shrinks it. In many women this is enough to stop troublesome symptoms, but if pain and heavy periods persist it may be necessary to consider surgery.

The final option for women with heavy periods is to have a hysterectomy. Though this may sound drastic, if you have found yourself organising your diary around when you are likely to be bleeding, or even avoiding making plans in case you are bleeding, it can give you a completely new lease of life.

HYSTERECTOMY

Eleanor, age 48

'My periods had got heavier and heavier over the past couple of years, but what was bothering me more was the pain. It was getting to the stage when I was finding it difficult to work – and on a couple of occasions I had to go off sick, which is completely not like me. So I thought I'd better see my doctor to get it sorted. She checked me over and said it felt like my womb was quite big, which explained why my jeans had been getting a bit tight – I'd just put it down to middle-aged spread. The scan she arranged showed that not only had I got several large fibroids, but that I'd also got a lot of adenomyosis – tissue like the lining of the womb, but inside the womb muscle – and that was why I was getting so much pain. I talked through my options with my doctor. As I was 46, she warned me I was likely to carry on having periods for another three or four years at least. I tried a Mirena, but though the pain and bleeding did ease a little, my tummy – and the fibroids – got bigger. So at 47 I decided to have a hysterectomy. I wasn't planning on having any more kids – my youngest was 10 – but even so I did feel that a vital part of me, as a woman, was being taken away, and I think that was the hardest bit to come to terms with. The surgery itself was OK – I was in hospital for three days, and needed six weeks off work, but once I recovered I felt so relieved that I didn't have to worry about pain and bleeding any more. My skin still bulges a bit above the scar, but overall my tummy is so much flatter, and more comfortable, than before.'

I understand entirely why women balk at the idea of losing their womb. After all, it is the place where an unborn baby grows, and for many it represents the very core of their femininity. Even if your family is complete, there is a world of difference between not wanting any more children and not being able to have any more children. That said, though, a woman's womb can cause her an awful lot of problems – not just heavy periods, but also pelvic pain and even urinary problems, and there are thousands of women who will testify that having their womb removed was the best thing they ever did.

Despite women's emotional attachment to their wombs, the uterus only has one biological function, and that is to incubate babies. It doesn't produce any hormones, and though the lining is shed once a month, that's only the body's response to the lack of a pregnancy. So removing the womb has just two consequences – you don't have periods and you can't bear a child. There is no change to your hormone levels, so you don't suddenly become menopausal, and neither should you suddenly pile on weight.

However, the continued cyclical production of hormones from the ovaries can mean you still get PMS, even though you don't have any periods. Your sex life should not be affected, as the vagina stays the same, and in fact many say their sex life improves, as they no longer suffer from heavy periods or pelvic pain, which previously interfered with lovemaking.

Things are rather different if the ovaries are removed as well. This is sometimes necessary if, for example, they are affected by endometriosis, or if they are stuck by adhesions (from previous inflammation) to the womb. If you are pre-, or perimenopausal, removing both ovaries results in a sudden fall in hormone levels and an abrupt menopause. If you are post-menopausal at the time of surgery, your ovaries will have already stopped working, so removing them shouldn't make any difference. You should always discuss beforehand with your gynaecologist about what is likely to happen to your ovaries – whether it is planned to leave them in place or remove them.

Unless you have cancer, the decision to have a hysterectomy should not be rushed, though it's probably easier for a woman to say goodbye to her womb in her late forties than it is for someone in their late thirties. It should be viewed as a last-resort option, when other alternative treatments are either unsuitable or have failed.

There are three main types of hysterectomy:

Abdominal hysterectomy. This involves removing the womb through a cut in the lower tummy wall, usually just below the top of the pubic hair line. The hair is shaved off before the operation, but when it grows back with luck the scar should be covered. Occasionally a vertical cut may be required straight down the lower abdomen, below the tummy button. Most women are discharged from hospital about four days after surgery. In most cases the womb, together with the cervix, is removed – a total abdominal hysterectomy, or TAH for short, but occasionally it is difficult to remove the cervix as well, so this is left behind – a 'subtotal hysterectomy'.

As with any form of major surgery, having a hysterectomy is not risk-free. Damage to the bladder or one of the ureters (the drainage tubes from the kidneys) occurs in about one in every 150 women having the operation, and much more rarely (about one in 2,500) there is damage to the bowel. Excessive bleeding during the operation means that about one in 50 women require a blood transfusion, and about one in 250 women develop a deep vein thrombosis afterwards. An infection may also occur in the wound.

Women who have had a subtotal hysterectomy may continue to have slight monthly bleeds afterwards, from the tissue lining the canal of the cervix. Because the cervix is still present, it is also important to continue to have regular smear tests. Women who have had the cervix removed do not normally need to continue having smears, unless the operation was done because of cervical cancer, or if smear tests were repeatedly abnormal beforehand.

Vaginal hysterectomy. This involves removing the womb through a cut in the top of the vagina. It involves the surgeon carefully cutting and tying the ligament and blood vessels that support and supply the womb – it's not done by suction, as I know some women believe. A vaginal hysterectomy has the advantage of not leaving any visible scars, and recovery is often much quicker, with some women being discharged from hospital two days after surgery. However, it's not suitable for all women – wombs that are enlarged by fibroids often cannot be removed this way – the hole in the top of the vagina simply can't be made big enough. Vaginal hysterectomy may be combined with a repair procedure to tighten up either the front or back wall of the vagina, or both. There is more information about this on page 266.

Like abdominal hysterectomy, there is a risk of damaging the bladder or ureters (this occurs in about one in 150 women) and a similar risk of bleeding. However, infection afterwards is less common.

Laparoscopic hysterectomy. Increasing numbers of hysterectomies are now being performed via keyhole surgery. This is done via three small incisions in the tummy wall, one on the edge of the tummy button, and one on either side of the lower tummy. It usually only involves a two- or three-day hospital stay, and recovery time is much quicker than with an abdominal hysterectomy. However, as with any keyhole surgery, it is important that it is performed by a surgeon specially trained and skilled in the method, to avoid possible complications such as accidental damage to the bladder or bowel. Even in the most skilled hands it is sometimes difficult for the womb to be removed via the laparoscope, and about one in 40 women have to have their tummy cut open in the conventional way for the operation to be completed.

GYNAECOLOGICAL CANCERS

No book about the menopause would be complete without a section on gynaecological cancer. Compared to breast cancer, they aren't common, but every woman should be aware of them and their symptoms. As with all cancers, early diagnosis can make a big difference to whether or not treatment is successful, and any women with concerns about symptoms should always see a doctor for a check-up. With ovarian cancer in particular, symptoms can be very vague, and far too many women are diagnosed with this at a late stage.

Ovarian cancer

This affects just under 7,000 women a year in the UK. The incidence is strongly related to age, and rises sharply in the late thirties. It's still rare before the menopause, though, and over three-quarters of cases are diagnosed in women aged 55 or over. Unlike breast cancer, the rate of ovarian cancer in the UK has fallen slightly in the last 10 years and this is probably related to use of the combined contraceptive pill, which reduces the risk slightly while it is taken and for 10 years afterwards.

As with so many cancers, anyone can be affected, but ovarian cancer is more common in women who have had a first-degree relative with the disease, especially at a young age, and those who carry BRCA1 or 2 genes are at increased risk of both ovarian and breast cancer, and also some types of bowel cancer. Screening for ovarian cancer, using ultrasound and blood tests, is now available for these women.

Women who have not had children, who start their periods early or who have late menopause, are also at slightly increased risk. A link has also been reported with the use of fertility drugs, but this seems to be confined to those who do not conceive – if the treatment is successful, there is no increased risk, so it may be the childlessness, rather than the fertility drugs per se that is the real risk.

Unfortunately, ovarian cancer is notorious for not causing any symptoms in the early stages. The telltale signs – a bloated abdomen, an increased need to pass urine or slight abdominal discomfort tend to only occur when the tumour has grown large, and even then the symptoms tend to be vague, so the diagnosis can be easily missed.

A pelvic examination may reveal an enlarged ovary, but the diagnosis is usually only suspected from a pelvic ultrasound scan, as cancerous cysts have a different appearance from benign ones. A raised blood level of the chemical CA125, which is produced by the cancer cells, also raises the suspicion of ovarian cancer.

Confirmation of the diagnosis can only be made by directly examining the ovary and removing the cyst. If cancer is confirmed, it is usual practice to remove the entire ovary, and often the other ovary and womb as well. Checking whether the cancer has spread – 'staging' – is done using either CT or MRI scans, and is used to determine what further treatment should be given. Most ovarian cancers respond, at least initially, to chemotherapy, usually a platinum-based drug, or Taxol or both.

If the disease is caught early, the outlook is good, and nine out of 10 women will be alive and well five years later. Unfortunately, if the diagnosis is made when the cancer has already spread (as is often the case) the overall outlook is less positive, and five-year survival rates are much lower.

Uterine cancer

There are two different types of cancer that affect the womb – cancer of the neck of the womb, or cervix, and cancer of the lining of the womb, endometrial cancer.

Endometrial cancer affects about 600 women a year in the UK. It is rare in pre-menopausal women, but in one in five it starts around the time of the menopause. It is most common in women aged 60 to 69.

Endometrial cancer is more common in women who have higher than average levels of unopposed oestrogen – that is, oestrogen that is not balanced by progesterone. Women who are overweight have an increased risk, as fat cells convert other hormones to small amounts of oestrogen, and there is also a slight increased risk in women who have had no children, or who have taken tamoxifen for treating or preventing breast cancer, or who have taken oestrogen-only HRT (though this practice should no longer happen). Women with BRCA1 and 2 genes are also slightly more at risk.

Unlike ovarian cancer, endometrial cancer usually causes symptoms fairly early, in the form of abnormal bleeding. In younger women this may be bleeding in between periods or, less commonly, prolonged, heavy periods. In women after the menopause it can be any bleeding – light spotting, or a slight bleed that occurs after sex, or more heavy bleeding – and this is why any vaginal bleeding that occurs after the menopause should always be checked out by your doctor.

An ultrasound scan can often reveal thickening of the womb lining, and the diagnosis is confirmed usually by a hysteroscopy and biopsy. Treatment commonly involves removing the whole womb, together with the ovaries, fallopian tubes and lymph nodes from the pelvis. For cancers that are caught in the early stages and are localised to the womb, this is the only treatment that is required. More advanced cancers which have spread may also require radiotherapy to the pelvic area, and additional chemotherapy may also be given to help stop further tumour growth.

As with so many cancers, the outlook depends on how early the cancer is diagnosed and treated. Because endometrial cancer tends to cause symptoms at an early stage, overall 74 per cent are alive and well after five years.

Cervical cancer affects just under 3,000 women each year in the UK. It is most commonly diagnosed in women aged 30 to 34, and unlike other cancers which become more common with increasing age, only 11 per cent of cases are diagnosed in women over 75.

Cervical cancer is caused by the human papilloma virus, usually referred to as HPV. There are more than 200 different strains of HPV. Around 40 of these are spread by sexual contact and some of these cause warts, while 15 other strains, which don't cause obvious warts, can cause the cellular changes that eventually lead to cancer. However, infection with HPV – which is virtually inevitable in a woman who is sexually active – may lead to only temporary change in the cells, which revert back to normal as the virus is cleared by the body's immune system. Cervical smear tests, which used to check for abnormal cells, are now changing to check for infection with high-risk strains of HPV. This is important, as in the past many women had unnecessary treatment for slight cellular abnormalities that would have reverted to normal naturally in the course of time.

The current guidelines in the UK are that women aged 25 to 49 should have a smear test once every three years and then once every five years between the ages of 50 and 64. Frequent smear tests in older women are not thought to be necessary as nearly all women in this age group will have become immune to HPV, and new changes will not occur in the cervical cells. Any woman who becomes newly sexually active at a later age should discuss with her GP whether she ought to have more frequent smear tests.

Teenage girls are now routinely offered vaccination against four strains of HPV virus that are known to cause the majority of cases of cervical cancer and genital warts, and hopefully this will mean that cervical cancer becomes less common in the future. However, having smear tests will remain important, as the vaccine does not provide protection against all cancer-inducing strains.

Treatment for an abnormal smear test depends on the degree of abnormality and whether high-risk HPV has been detected. For those with the infection, and persistent abnormal cells, the usual treatment is to destroy the abnormal cells with heat (either electrical diathermy or a laser). If abnormal cells extend up the cervical canal, removing them surgically – a cone biopsy – may be necessary.

Cervical cancer only tends to occur in women who have not had a smear test for many years, and often not at all. Symptoms can include abnormal bleeding, especially after sex, plus a vaginal discharge. The cervix usually has an abnormal appearance when examined, and the diagnosis can be confirmed by a smear test together with a biopsy. Treatment usually involves removing the womb, the ovaries and the surrounding pelvic lymph nodes, often followed by radiotherapy. As with all cancers, outlook depends on how quickly the disease is diagnosed and treated, Overall, two-thirds of women with cervical cancer survive for five years or more.

Vulval cancer

This affects around 1,200 women a year in the UK. It is strongly linked with HPV infection, and women who have had a moderate to severe change in a smear test or who have had cervical cancer have up to a 10 times increased risk of vulval cancer. Unlike cervical cancer, though, the risk of vulval cancer increases with age, with the peak incidence being aged 65 to 69. The risk is increased by smoking, and there is also a slightly increased risk in women with the skin condition lichen sclerosus, especially if it has not been treated adequately.

Symptoms of vulval cancer can include a persistent lump or ulcer, which is painful when urine touches it, and soreness. Occasionally there may be itching. A biopsy needs to be taken for diagnosis. Treatment involves surgery to remove the cancerous area with a large margin of normal tissue, and it may be necessary to remove the surrounding lymph nodes as well. A combination of radiotherapy and chemotherapy may be required to stop further spread in some patients. As symptoms tend to occur early, the outlook is good, and overall, around 60 per cent of women with vulval cancer will survive 5 years or more.

CASE HISTORIES

Lorraine, age 49

HER STORY: My periods were fairly regular until a few months ago. Then I missed one, and a couple of weeks after that, I suddenly had the most horrendous heavy bleed. It was like having a miscarriage, only I can't have been pregnant because I haven't had sex for ages. I just had to sit on the loo – there was no way I could get into work. Then it happened again six weeks later – same pattern – a sudden really heavy bleed which tailed off after a few days. I can't keep taking days off work – what can I do about this? And how long is it going to continue?

MY ADVICE: I explained that this sounded like 'anovulatory' cycles. Her ovaries were still producing some oestrogen, which was causing a build-up in the womb lining, but she wasn't ovulating, and therefore wasn't producing any progesterone, which normally balances the effects of oestrogen on the womb lining. Eventually the oestrogen-thickened endometrium becomes unstable and breaks down, causing a horrendous heavy flow of blood. However, it was important to do some tests to check that there wasn't another reason for her heavy bleeds, so I did a pelvic examination (which was normal) and arranged for her to have a pelvic ultrasound scan, to rule out fibroids or a structural abnormality in her pelvis. I also arranged blood tests which showed that though her thyroid hormone levels were normal, her haemoglobin was at the low end of normal, and her iron level was low. This meant that her heavy bleeds were depleting her body of iron faster than she was making it up through her intake from her diet, and if this pattern continued she would become anaemic. I also checked her FSH level, which was 18, suggesting she was perimenopausal.

There was no easy way of predicting if she was going to continue having erratic heavy bleeds. It was possible they could continue for another six months, or alternatively, that she wouldn't have any more.

I suggested her options were to have a supply of tranexamic acid, which she could start taking as soon as another bleed started. I also suggested that if she wanted I could fit a Mirena coil. However, the disadvantage of this was that it could take several months to 'settle' into her womb, and that during this time she might have continuous bleeding. As she was already perimenopausal, I didn't think the combined pill was a good choice for her, as her periods might stop any day – and if she went on the Pill she wouldn't know what was happening to her own body. If she needed contraception it might have been more of an appropriate option, but she didn't currently have a partner, and she said if she did meet someone, she would insist they use a condom (sensible woman!).

She opted for tranexamic acid. She did have another couple of bleeds, but the pills made the flow lighter, which meant she was able to get into work. Then her periods stopped, but she admitted she felt she couldn't really relax and go out without protection until she had a year free of any bleeding.

Melissa, age 50

HER STORY: My periods are all over the place. They're not too heavy – if anything they are lighter than normal – it's just I never know when I'm going to have one, and in my job that's a real problem. I can be stuck in a long meeting and suddenly can feel I've started bleeding. I've taken to wearing a pad all the time. I'm also getting hot flushes and sweats, and feeling tired. What is the best thing to do? Would HRT help?

MY ADVICE: This type of bleeding pattern is very common at the menopause. It is difficult to predict how long it will continue, but it is unusual for it to continue for more than a year. There was nothing in Melissa's story that concerned me as suggesting anything was seriously wrong. The fact that she was having flushes and sweats meant that her oestrogen production was falling, and therefore the chances were that her periods would stop fairly soon. I explained that one option was to do nothing, and just wait and see how things went for the next couple of months. However, she said the flushes and sweats were becoming a real nuisance, and she'd like to do something about them, and that would hopefully help her bleeding as well. I explained that HRT could stop her flushes within a few days, but the erratic bleeding might continue. She opted to give it a try anyway, and chose tablets, which she would find easy to take. It took six months to find an HRT that suited her, as initially she got a lot of headaches and bloating. However, on the third regime, a combination of 1mg estradiol with an additional 1mg norethisterone for 12 days each month, she felt OK. Her flushes and sweats were much reduced and she was only getting bleeding at the end of the norethisterone tablets, which was possibly because her own ovaries had ceased to function altogether. The only way to know this would be for her to stop the HRT, but as that would mean a sudden return of her flushes and sweats, she decided not to bother.

Rosie, age 47

HER STORY: My periods have always been a bit painful, but recently they are much worse, though they are still regular. And they are heavier, too – I sometimes have to wear a tampon and a pad. Sex has been a bit uncomfortable sometimes, too. Is this the menopause?

MY ADVICE: This didn't sound like the menopause, but rather something else causing her to have heavy, painful periods. The possibilities were a pelvic infection, fibroids, endometriosis or adenomyosis. When I did a pelvic examination, there was no sign of any discharge (making an infection unlikely), and the swabs I took all came back negative. However, her womb felt slightly larger than normal, and she found the examination uncomfortable. Though an ultrasound scan is not a good way of diagnosing endometriosis outside the womb, in Rosie's case it showed a difference in the consistency of the wall of her womb, suggesting adenomyosis.

I discussed possible treatment options with her. As she was 47, she was likely to be having periods for another three years, so I recommended she have a Mirena fitted. This would reduce the amount of adenomyosis tissue present in her womb, and within about six months should make her periods lighter and less painful. It could also stay in place for five years, so would also help with any erratic heavy bleeding that might occur around the time of the menopause.

She went along with this suggestion, and though she had a lot of bleeding for the first two months after it was fitted, her periods did gradually become lighter, and though she still had some pain on the first day of her period, it was much less than before.

Anne, age 48

HER STORY: I've had some bleeding in between my periods and it's also started happening a bit after sex as well. To begin with I thought it was the start of the change, but then I realised I haven't had a smear test for ages, and I'm a bit worried. Is this the menopause, or could it be anything serious?

MY ADVICE: Bleeding like this in between periods, and after sex, cannot be blamed on the menopause. First of all she needed a pelvic examination, and this revealed a small polyp coming out of the middle of her cervix. I took a smear test, which came back showing no abnormal cells. An ultrasound scan showed that the polyp actually originated in her womb, and was quite large, so she needed to be referred to the local gynaecology clinic. She had a hysteroscopy under a brief anaesthetic and the polyp was removed.

Janine, age 46

HER STORY: My periods have gradually got heavier and heavier. They are now lasting at least 10 days, often longer. I sometimes only have about a week each month when I'm not bleeding. I'm also having to get up at night to go to the loo, and go more often during the day, so I think I must have got a urinary infection. Are the two connected? Am I approaching the menopause?

MY ADVICE: Though it was possible that the change in her bleeding pattern was due to a change in her hormone levels, I was suspicious that her womb was enlarged and pressing on her bladder, which was why she was needing to go to the loo more often. When I examined her abdomen, I could feel that her uterus was much larger than normal, reaching halfway to her tummy button. An ultrasound scan confirmed that she had several large fibroids.

We discussed treatment and she was keen to avoid having surgery if possible, so to begin with she had a trial of ulipristal, taking a tablet a day for three months. Her fibroids did shrink slightly, but she continued to need to go to the toilet frequently, had quite a lot of headaches during the treatment and did not want to take a further course. She reluctantly decided that as she was only 46, and had another three or four years of periods ahead of her, the best course of action was surgery. As her womb was still quite large, her gynaecologist recommended that she had a course of GnRH injections, to try to shrink it further. This made it possible for her to have her womb removed laparoscopically, so she avoided having a large scar. And as only her womb was removed, she did not go through an instant menopause and made a very quick recovery afterwards.

SUMMARY

📖 The menstrual cycle always changes in the approach to the menopause, but exactly want happens can vary enormously.

📖 Some women find that their periods just become more irregular, and lighter.

📖 Others are not nearly so lucky and have very erratic bleeds, which may be incredibly heavy.

📖 It can be difficult to predict how long the 'menstrual chaos' that can occur at the menopause will last, and though an occasional heavy period may be nothing to worry about, if it happens repeatedly it can, and often does, lead to iron-deficiency anaemia.

- Other gynaecological problems often occur in women in their forties, such as fibroids. It is important not to assume all changes in bleeding are just due to the approach of the menopause.

- Effective treatments are available that can help with heavy, erratic periods, so do not hesitate to get medical advice.

8

....

SEX

There are two rather different sides to the topic of sex and the menopause.

Firstly, for women approaching the menopause, is the issue of whether or not contraception is still needed and, if so, what is the best method to use. Then there is the issue of sex after the menopause. On the plus side, you don't need to worry about contraception or an unwanted pregnancy any more, but on the negative side, libido has a habit of going through the floor and sex just drops off the agenda of things that seem even remotely important. If you do want to have sex, the arousal response seems to have disappeared and your vagina stays dry, making intercourse uncomfortable, even if you are with the man of your dreams.

So this chapter is divided into two halves; the first giving advice on contraception – how long you need to use it for, and the most suitable methods for perimenopausal women. Then there is a section for post-menopausal women – how to maintain an enjoyable sex life. There are some real-life case histories at the end, but I'll start with the common questions that women would like answered.

I really don't want children at this time in my life. How long do I need to continue using contraception?

The standard advice to this question is until a year after your last period. The ovaries wind down in an erratic fashion, and theoretically at least you could still ovulate a few months after your periods appear to have stopped. In practice, your eggs are so old by now, biologically speaking, that if one was fertilised it's likely not to develop properly, which makes you much more likely to have a miscarriage or a baby with a genetic defect. Using contraception that prevents a pregnancy is a far better option.

Is it safe to take the combined pill up until the menopause?

For many women, yes. It all depends on other factors that affect your general health. The combined pill contains synthetic oestrogen and progesterone in much higher doses than those found in HRT. In general it's the oestrogen that can cause problems for slightly older women, as this can increase the risk of blood clots and strokes. For instance, if you are a smoker, overweight, have high blood pressure, diabetes or bad migraines, you shouldn't be taking the Pill in your late forties. But if you are otherwise in good health, it can be a good option, especially as it can help to stop the menstrual chaos that can occur around the time of the change.

What about the mini-pill? Or the implant?

These only contain synthetic progestogens, which have fewer serious side effects than oestrogen. Both can be used by most women right up until the menopause, and can be a good option for women who can't take the combined pill. However, unlike the combined pill, they may not stop the heavy, erratic periods that can occur in the perimenopause.

I've got a Mirena coil and don't have any periods. When will I know that I'm going through the change? When should I have it removed?

The simple answer to when will you know is – with difficulty! Flushes and sweats may be a giveaway that you are approaching the change, but not all women get these. A hormone test for FSH levels can be helpful. In practice, a Mirena coil lasts for five years, and I usually recommend that women leave it in for this time. Unless it is causing problems, there is no need to remove it any earlier, and if you want to take HRT, for either menopausal symptoms or to protect your bones, you only need oestrogen as the progestogen from the coil protects the womb lining.

I used to really enjoy a good sex life with my husband, but since my periods stopped, I really couldn't care less about it any more. Is this normal?

Unfortunately, yes. The lack of hormone production from the ovaries, especially oestrogen and testosterone, usually causes a very unwelcome fall in libido after the menopause. HRT can boost up oestrogen levels, and usually goes some way to help maintain libido. If you don't want, or can't take HRT, then the alternative, boosting testosterone is much more difficult. Many couples find a way round a woman's lack of libido, but it certainly helps to be in a good relationship with an understanding partner.

I'm in my mid-fifties, and after my divorce, I'm dating again. But I'm finding it difficult to get aroused, even with men I really fancy. Why is this and what can I do about it?

It's all to do with the drop in oestrogen. This helps to keep the tissues in the genital area moist and plump, and also drives an increase in the production of lubricating fluids in response to sexual arousal. After the menopause the genital area usually becomes much more dry, and the labia shrink slightly. Applying oestrogen directly to the genital tissues can be very helpful in reversing these post-menopausal changes, and can be done either using cream or pessaries. Using a lubricating gel just before sex can also be helpful. Those based on oils, rather than water, are best, but be careful if you are using condoms, as some oils can damage latex.

CONTRACEPTION IN THE PERIMENOPAUSE

In theory, it's possible to become pregnant even if you are only ovulating sporadically, and for this reason it's recommended that if you don't want a baby, you should use contraception for a year after your last natural period. And that's what I always recommend to my patients.

It's a myth to think that just because you are in your mid-forties you can't get pregnant, and that it's OK to have unprotected sex. In 2013 over 7,600 abortions were performed in women aged between 40 and 44, 686 in women aged 45 to 49, and 24 in those over 50. Proof that older women can still be fertile, and need to use contraception!

Once you are in your late forties the eggs that are being produced are of much lower quality than before, and even if one is successfully fertilised, the chances of the embryo developing into a normal healthy baby are slim. Chromosome abnormalities, with some extra, or some missing, are extremely common, and often incompatible with life. That means that if you do get pregnant in your late forties, the chances are higher that you will have a miscarriage. No one wants that, so it really is better to take precautions to stop a pregnancy occurring in the first place.

So what are the options for contraception for women in their forties? In most cases, the choice is as wide as it is for much younger women, but some methods do have to be used with a bit more care.

There are two main types of contraception – those that contain hormones, and those that don't. In general, hormonal methods are best for what you want contraception to do, which is preventing you from getting pregnant. They also can be very good at controlling the menstrual chaos that can occur around the time of the menopause. However, they are the worst for side effects, and they don't offer any protection against sexually transmitted infections. Just because you are older does not make you immune to these and, in fact, the number of cases of sexually transmitted infections (STIs) is growing at an alarming rate in women over 40 – mainly because they are not taking any precautions against them.

HORMONAL METHODS

These can be divided into two groups: those that contain oestrogen- and progesterone-like hormones (so-called 'combined methods') and those that contain progesterone alone.

Frannie, age 51

'I stopped taking the Pill after my divorce in my early forties. A couple of years later I started dating again, and to begin with used condoms, but I hated them, and when I settled with my new partner, we didn't bother to use anything. I honestly thought I was too old to get pregnant. It was on my forty-sixth birthday that I found out I was expecting. It was a horrible shock. I decided to have a termination, and sitting in the waiting room with all the young girls at the clinic, I felt so embarrassed and ashamed. Afterwards I went through my contraceptive options with the nurse at the surgery – I couldn't bring myself to see my doctor, I felt so stupid. I wanted something that was really reliable, but didn't fancy having a coil. She said I could go back to the Pill – which surprised me at my age. But I didn't smoke, and had no health problems, and I'd never had a problem forgetting to take it. It's worked well for me. I have to watch my weight carefully – but that would probably happen at my age anyway – my periods are lighter than before and, better still, I can alter their timing so I never have one when I'm going away.'

Combined methods

These include the Pill, the patch and the ring. All these methods contain two hormones: one based on oestrogen and another based on progesterone. The amount of oestrogen in contraceptives is far higher than the amount used in HRT, and is enough to suppress the natural cycle and stop the ovaries working, so that ovulation does not occur. The progesterone component alters the mucus at the entrance to the womb (which helps to prevent sperm entry) and also the womb lining, so in the unlikely event of an egg being released, it is rare that it will be fertilised or implant into the womb.

The good ...

One big advantage of combined methods, especially for perimenopausal women, is that they give regular periods, which are also lighter and less painful than before. Premenstrual symptoms are also reduced, along with mood swings and other problems that are linked with the fluctuations of hormones that occur in a natural cycle.

And the bad ...

Side effects are an important consideration, especially in slightly older women. The oestrogen they contain can increase the risk of venous blood clots – deep vein thrombosis – and the tendency for oestrogen to increase blood pressure can be a nuisance, especially for older women. If you are over 40 and your blood pressure is greater than 135/85, combined methods are not for you. Unlike HRT, oestrogen-containing contraceptives cannot be used together with medication to reduce blood pressure. The dose of oestrogen is just too high.

The oestrogen in combined methods can also increase the risk of stroke, and all these three major risks increase with age, by being overweight and also by smoking. If you are medically obese with a Body Mass Index of over 30, or you smoke, you can't have oestrogen-containing contraceptives if you are 35 or over. But if you don't smoke, are not overweight and have no other risk factors (which include diabetes, severe migraines or a history of gallstones) you can use oestrogen-containing contraceptives right up until the menopause.

One other important consideration, though, is breast cancer. The oestrogen in the Pill increases, very slightly, the risk of breast cancer.

This means that it's not suitable for women who have had breast cancer, and those who could be at increased risk due to a family history of the disease should, in my view, try other methods first.

Another drawback of any contraceptives containing oestrogen is that they can stimulate the growth of fibroids. This usually doesn't matter with small fibroids, but it can make moderate or large fibroids more likely to cause symptoms.

Less serious, but sometimes just as troubling, side effects can include nausea (especially when the method is first started), tender breasts and slight weight gain. You may find you need a larger bra cup size and fighting middle-aged spread is just a little bit more difficult.

Another issue – disguising the menopause

One of the issues for older women taking combined methods is that it can make it very difficult to know whether you are menopausal or not. The monthly bleeds that occur are not natural periods, but rather a withdrawal bleed that occurs when hormones are stopped for a week each month. In most women the ovaries do start producing hormones again within a day or so of stopping using the pill (or the patch or ring) but if the ovaries have stopped working the sudden drop in hormones can lead to hot flushes and sweats in the hormone-free week. But many women have no idea if they are menopausal or not until they stop using extra hormones for at least a couple of weeks. Not only this, but blood tests to check for FSH levels while you are using oestrogen-containing contraceptives are useless, simply because the external oestrogen suppresses the production of FSH. Blood tests are really only accurate once you have stopped using oestrogen for at least a month, which gives time for the pituitary gland to recover from any effects of external oestrogen. In itself, this doesn't really matter – there is no harm in carrying on taking the Pill until you are 50, but it can make it impossible to know when it's safe to stop using contraception. It just has to be a case of 'try it and see what happens'.

Factor V Leiden

Factor V Leiden is an abnormal type of the protein factor V, which is required for blood clotting. It's an inherited condition caused by a gene defect and affects around 5 per cent of the population. Those who inherit the gene from one parent ('heterozygous') have an eight-time risk of thrombosis compared to others, while those who inherit it from both parents ('homozygous') have up to 130 times increased risk. Testing can be done via a blood sample and a thrombophilia screen. Carrying Factor V Leiden is also linked with an increased risk of recurrent miscarriage, caused by tiny clots within the blood vessels supplying the developing foetus. Anyone with a family history of blood clots or miscarriage can request a test from their GP. Those with Factor V Leiden should not use contraceptives containing oestrogen and should also avoid using HRT if possible.

Which combined method?

Pills

The most popular, by far, of the combined methods is the Pill. There are lots of different combinations of hormones available, and though in the past the Pill was usually prescribed by a brand name, such as Microgynon or Yasmin, now it is prescribed by the names of the individual hormone ingredients. Several different brands have identical contents, so this can mean that you get pills with different brand names each time you pick up your prescription from the chemist.

Most pills contain the same oestrogen, ethinyl oestradiol, usually in a dose of 30mcg, though some have 35mcg, and a couple of 'low-dose' pills have 20mcg. The type and amount of progesterone is more variable, and it is very much the progesterone component and the balance with oestrogen that can make a pill more suitable for an individual woman than another. Pills that are relatively more oestrogenic are more likely to cause bloating, weight gain and nausea, while those that are more progestogenic tend to be more suitable for women who tend to have very heavy periods but are more likely to cause acne, depression and greasy skin. Generally, it's a question of 'try it and see', but it can take three months for your body to get used to a hormone mix, so even if it doesn't at first seem suitable, try not to give up on each brand too soon.

One big advantage of taking the combined pill is that you can predict, to the day, when you are going to have a period. That's great at any age, but particularly in the perimenopausal years when your cycle can go completely haywire. Better still, if your period is due to start at an inconvenient time – for instance, when you are about to go off on holiday – you can simply take two packets in a row without a break. You can also do this regularly if you have awful heavy periods – there's no need to have a monthly bleed if you don't want one – once every two to three months is fine, though withdrawal bleeds after six weeks of pill-taking are likely to be more heavy than after three weeks.

The patch

Like the combined pill, this contains both oestrogen and progesterone. The big difference is that instead of swallowing the hormones by mouth, they are absorbed through the skin. The patch only needs changing once a week, so it's ideal for women who find it difficult to remember to take a pill every day. The patch is worn for three weeks, then there is a 'patch-free week' when a withdrawal bleed, like a period, occurs (just like the Pill). But like all patch medicines, the adhesive can irritate sensitive skins and leave an annoying line of glue when it's removed. The patch is suitable and not suitable for the same groups of women as the Pill, and the side effects are the same. The patch is more expensive than the Pill, which means that some doctors and family planning clinics may be reluctant to prescribe it, but as with all slightly more expensive methods, this is a bit of a nonsense, as it's a lot cheaper than dealing with an unwanted pregnancy (and that's the argument you need to use if necessary!).

The vaginal ring

This is a flexible, see-through ring, just over 5cm in diameter, which contains two hormones – again, just like the combined pill. It is inserted into the vagina, from where the hormones are absorbed, and left in place for three weeks. Then there is a hormone-free week, when the monthly withdrawal bleed occurs. Theoretically the ring can be left in place during sex, but it may be more comfortable for your partner if it's removed. However, it needs to be put back in as soon as possible, and certainly within three hours, and it shouldn't be removed frequently or it becomes less effective (fewer hormones are absorbed). If you have any bleeding while the ring is in place it is fine to use tampons. Side effects are the same as with the combined pill, plus also it may cause a vaginal discharge and a sore vagina. Overall, my view of the ring is it's worth considering if you want the benefits of a combined hormone method, are not good at remembering daily pills and have a sensitive skin.

Progesterone-only methods

Lottie, age 46

'My third child, at the age of 42, was what I think is called a "happy accident". I hadn't been planning on having any more kids, and I was taking the progesterone-only pill. Only I wasn't taking it, not properly. I kept forgetting it, not deliberately. I'd only realise when I did remember to take it that I'd missed a couple of days. So after Ellie was born, I thought I'd better be a bit more responsible and accept that taking pills was not a good idea for me. Even with the best will in the world, with my lifestyle and three young kids, I was bound to forget one sooner or later. My doctor mentioned the implant, but advised that the coil would give my body less hormones and so less side effects. The fitting was uncomfortable and I had cramps, like period pains, for several hours afterwards. And I also had bleeding, on and off, for the next two months. But since then, it's been great. My periods are so light, I only have to wear a panty liner for a couple of days. I don't have to think about contraception on a day-to-day basis, but rather I can forget about it for the next five years.'

Several different types of contraception are based on synthetic progesterone (progestogens):

- The progesterone-only pill – often called the POP or sometimes the 'mini-pill'

- Intrauterine systems, or coils

- Implants

- Injections.

Progestogens work as contraceptives by altering the environment in the cervix and womb, making it hostile to sperm – they simply die off before they reach and fertilise the egg. However, this effect is short-lived, and if levels fall the mucus and womb lining rapidly return to normal. So for progestogen methods to be effective, there has to be a constant supply of the hormone. Low doses of progestogens don't stop ovulation, but higher doses (such as those found in the implant and injection) can. This increases contraceptive efficiency, but as always the downside is more problems with unwanted side effects.

The good ...

Progestogen methods can be used by women of all ages, right up until the menopause, including those who can't use methods containing oestrogen. So they are suitable for older women who are overweight, have high blood pressure, or who are at increased risk of a DVT.

And the bad ...

Side effects can include a greasy skin and acne, though this is generally only an issue for women who have a tendency towards this anyway. Other side effects can include weight gain, headaches, mood changes (such as depression) and loss of libido.

Which method?

The Pill

There are several different brands of progesterone-only pill (POP) available, but by far the most popular is the one containing the progestogen desogestrel. This is because, unlike the others, it does tend to stop ovulation and so is more effective as a contraceptive. However, it's not quite as effective as the combined pill – one or two women in every hundred users will accidentally fall pregnant in a year, and that's when it's being taken properly. As with the combined pill, forgetting pills makes the method less effective. Unlike the combined pill, the POP has to be taken every day, without a break. The most troublesome side effect of this pill method is erratic periods, sometimes with bleeding in between them. If you need to know when you are going to have a period, this method is not for you. It will also not control the chaotic bleeding that can occur around the time of the menopause.

The intra-uterine system, or IUS

This looks like a T-shaped coil and, like other coils, has to be inserted into the womb. What makes it very different to other coils is that instead of having fine copper wire on the stem, there is a sheath of progestogen. A small amount of this is released continually, right where it's needed, inside the womb. This makes it highly effective as a contraceptive – better than the combined pill and, surprisingly, more effective than being sterilised. No method can claim to be 100 per cent effective, but if you have an IUS fitted, particularly the higher-dose one, you are very, very unlikely to accidentally fall pregnant.

There are two versions: the Mirena and its slightly smaller little sister, the Jaydess. The Mirena can stay in place for five years, the Jaydess for three. Both release a tiny amount of progestogen each day, and only a small fraction of this reaches the general circulation, meaning that unwanted side effects, such as greasy skin or weight gain, are far less likely to occur.

One huge advantage of the IUS is that once it has settled in, periods become very light indeed and sometimes completely disappear. This is simply because the womb lining is so thin there is nothing to come away, and the Mirena is now used regularly as a treatment for heavy periods. It is also extremely good at controlling the heavy periods that can occur around the time of the menopause. Better still, it can be used as the 'progestogen' part of HRT, so if you do get flushes and sweats, and have a Mirena in place, all you need to take is oestrogen. You don't need progesterone pills as well.

The Jaydess is a more recent introduction and is mainly aimed at younger women. One reason for this is that the Mirena can be slightly painful to fit, especially in women who have never been pregnant, who tend to have a very narrow canal through the cervix into the womb. At the time of writing, the Jaydess is only licensed for use as a contraceptive, not for treating heavy periods or for use with HRT. Both devices have two tiny nylon threads that come out through the cervix, which mean that you can check it's in place, and they are also the means by which the device is removed. As long as these have been trimmed by the fitter to the right length, your partner should not be able to feel these during sex. As with all coils, the IUS cannot move once it has been fitted – the rare stories you may read about coils being found in the abdominal cavity occur because they have accidentally been put there during the fitting, with the fitter pushing the device into the womb too hard, so that a hole is made in the wall of the womb. Needless to say, this really shouldn't happen.

With both the Mirena and the Jaydess, erratic bleeding can occur in the first few months after fitting, so it's not a good idea to have one fitted just before you jet off on holiday. But overall the IUS is a fantastic choice for women in the run-up to the menopause.

Implants

The implant is a very small flexible tube, 40mm long, containing progestogen which is inserted under the skin of the upper arm. A small amount of hormone is continually released – enough to stop ovulation as well as thickening the mucus at the neck of the womb. This makes it an extremely effective contraceptive, and fewer than one woman in a thousand who have one fitted will get pregnant in a year. It lasts up to three years, when it needs to be removed and replaced. The biggest disadvantage of the implant is that erratic bleeding can occur, especially in the first year after fitting, which may be prolonged. Some women, though, have very light, infrequent periods. Generally, the Mirena is a better choice for the perimenopausal woman.

Injections

These contain a progestogen which is injected into muscles, usually the buttock, from where it is slowly released. There are three different ones available in the UK, one which lasts 13 weeks, one eight, and the most popular, Depo-Provera, which lasts 12 weeks. Like the implant, they are highly effective. However, the dose of progestogen they contain is quite high, and this can make side effects, such as acne and weight gain, more of a problem. Not great if you are already struggling with the beginnings of middle-age spread. Erratic bleeding, which can be heavy and continuous, can also be a problem in the first six months of use, though after this periods may completely disappear. Injections tend to suppress the normal ovarian function, which means that not only does ovulation not occur (which makes it a good contraceptive) but oestrogen levels are lowered, too. This in turn can affect bone density, therefore injections are not a good idea for older women in their forties who may already be at increased risk of osteoporosis.

Barrier methods

Freya, age 53

'My body just didn't seem to be suited to having extra hormones. I must have tried about 10 different types of pill – with either both oestrogen or oestrogen and progesterone – and either I got headaches, weight gain or mood swings, or I lost my sex drive. I tried the Mirena coil but just like the progesterone pill I piled on weight, even though my doctor kept trying to tell me that the hormone dose to my body was really low. My husband hated using condoms, so I tried using a cap. I got on OK with it, but there was no doubt it was a bit intrusive – just when we were working up to having sex I'd have to go to the bathroom to get the thing in. And a couple of times when I came back to bed my hubby had dropped off to sleep! So I decided to give the copper coil a try. My periods have been heavier since it was put in, and overall they last around nine to 10 days, as I have some brown sludgy bleeding at the beginning and end of every period. But for me, it's the best option.'

Barrier methods aim to work by preventing any sperm reaching inside the womb or fallopian tubes, so that any egg that has been released cannot be fertilised.

The good ...

Though they are not quite as effective as hormonal methods for preventing pregnancies, these have the big advantage of providing protection against sexually transmitted infections and should therefore be used by all women, pre- and post-menopause, if you are with a new partner. They can also be an excellent method of contraception when you are having infrequent sex, and can be useful for older women with lower fertility when the risk of an unwanted pregnancy is lower. And, of course, the lack of hormones means you do know exactly what is happening to your natural cycle and when your periods are stopping of their own accord.

The bad ...

Failure rates are higher than with hormonal methods. Even with perfect use, between four and eight women out of 100 each year will accidentally become pregnant, and if not used correctly the failure rates are much higher.

Condoms are available for women as well as men, though many do report that it is a bit like using a bin liner in your vagina. **Diaphragms** are made of rubber and are between 60 and 90mm wide, and these sit along the front wall of the vagina covering the cervix. To get it in the right place takes a bit of practice, but once you are used to it they can be remarkably easy to insert and remove. **Caps** cover just the cervix, and are more fiddly, and for this reason are falling out of favour. Both caps and diaphragms should be used with spermicide, and can be put in place up to two hours before sex, then they must be left in place for a minimum of six hours afterwards. Neither should interfere with sex in any way.

The biggest problem with diaphragms is often finding a doctor who is skilled at fitting them – you may need to go to a family planning clinic rather than rely on your local GP.

Copper coils – the IUCD

Like the hormone-containing coil, these are small T-shaped pieces of plastic, about 1.5cm long, that are placed inside the womb. Instead of a hormone sheath, a fine coil of copper wire is wound round the stem. The exact way they work isn't known, but it's thought they interfere with the way sperm swim up through the cervix and the inside of the womb, preventing them reaching the egg. If an egg is fertilised, it may also prevent it implanting in the womb.

The good ...

Failure rates are between 1 and 2 per cent – not as good as the Mirena, but better than barrier methods. Depending on the device used, and your age, a copper coil can stay in place for between five and seven years, and up to 10 years in women in their forties. So it's good for long-term contraception, especially in older women.

The bad ...

The big disadvantage of copper coils is that they usually make periods heavy and more prolonged. That's OK if you usually have fairly light periods, but not if your periods are becoming heavier, especially around the time of the menopause. There is also a risk, albeit extremely small, that if an egg is fertilised when a copper coil is in place, it is more likely to lodge in the fallopian tube – an ectopic pregnancy. My view is that if you want an intra-uterine device you are far better off having a Mirena, especially in your forties, unless you really don't want to use any hormones.

Sterilisation

Arabella, age 48

'I seemed to get pregnant at the drop of a hat. Though my first two kids were planned, I fell for them as soon as I stopped the Pill, and my last two were accidents. I was on the Pill, and I did try to take it regularly, but I did forget it on a few occasions. I reckon my husband and I were super-fertile – I knew other couples who had taken far more risks than us and hadn't ended up with another baby. Four kids was enough, and we decided that we needed to do something to make sure our family didn't get any bigger. I had a Mirena coil fitted, but at times sex was more uncomfortable, and my husband said he could feel the strings. So we talked about sterilisation. Our doctor explained it was easier for my husband to 'be done' and, unlike some of his mates, the thought of 'firing blanks' didn't bother him at all. The op was done one morning in the local hospital outpatient clinic, under a local anaesthetic, and though he was quite bruised afterwards, he was out playing with the kids later the same day. It took six months before the sperm cleared from his semen, and we waited until he'd had two clear tests before I had the coil removed. We know it's not reversible, and that we'll not have any more kids, but for us, that's fine.'

Both men and women can be sterilised, and the idea is that you are then permanently unable to have children. You might think this would be a good solution for older couples in their forties, who are absolutely sure they do not want to have any more children, but drawbacks in the methods for both men and women, and the advent of the Mirena device, mean it's not as popular as it used to be.

Female sterilisation methods are based on blocking the fallopian tubes, so that the sperm can't reach the egg. There are two methods: the more traditional approach, laparoscopic sterilisation, involves keyhole surgery under a general anaesthetic, and clips or rings being placed around the fallopian tubes.

The newer method, hysteroscopic sterilisation, is done under local anaesthetic and involves a small tube with a camera attached being passed up through the cervix into the womb. A tiny implant is then placed inside the entrance to each fallopian tube, which stimulates the growth of scar tissue, which then blocks the tube. This process takes three months, and you should use another form of contraception until you have had a special X-ray done of the inside of the womb, using dye, to confirm the tubes are blocked.

Both methods are equally effective, but neither is foolproof. Around five women out of 1,000 will become pregnant after being sterilised, a higher failure rate than the Mirena. Reversing female sterilisation is extremely difficult, and pregnancies afterwards are rare, but if you are in your forties and all other methods are unsuitable – and I'm aware that this applies to a surprising number of women – sterilisation can be a good option.

Male sterilisation, a vasectomy, involves cutting the tubes that carry sperm from the testes to the penis. The procedure itself is more straightforward than in women, and is done under local anaesthetic, via a tiny cut on each side of the groin, beside the top of the scrotum. It doesn't work instantly, as it can take between three and six months for all sperm to disappear from the ejaculate, and other contraception is required until two semen tests have confirmed no live sperm are present. Sperm only make up a tiny amount of semen, and there is usually no noticeable difference in the ejaculate afterwards. Neither is there any increased risk of prostate cancer afterwards.

Emergency contraception

There are two ways you can stop yourself becoming pregnant after having unprotected sex.

The pill method

There are two kinds, one containing the progestogen levonorgestrel, and the other containing the hormone ulipristal. The levonorgestrel pill is thought to work by either delaying ovulation or by preventing the fertilised egg implanting in the womb. It can be taken up to 72 hours after unprotected sex, but is most effective if taken as soon as possible. If taken within 24 hours, 95 per cent of pregnancies are prevented, but if delayed for between 50 and 72 hours, it is only 58 per cent effective.

The ulipristal pill works mainly by delaying ovulation, but also has an effect on the lining of the womb. It can be taken up to 120 hours (five days) after unprotected sex. It too is more effective the sooner it is taken, but overall it is more effective than the levonorgestrel pill.

Both are available on prescription, and the levonorgestrel pill can also be purchased directly from pharmacies. Neither should be viewed as a substitute for pre-sex contraception, but they are certainly better than nothing, and unless you are using a long-term method, it's a good idea to keep an emergency pill in your medicine cupboard, right up until a year after your periods stop. You never know when you might need it.

The coil method

A copper IUCD can help protect against pregnancy after unprotected sex up to five days after the expected date of ovulation. If you have a regular 28-day cycle, you will expect to ovulate on day 14, meaning that a coil can be put in up until day 19 of your cycle, regardless of when you had sex. It can also be used after multiple episodes of unprotected sex. It's more effective than the emergency pill at preventing a pregnancy after unprotected sex, and has the advantage that it can be left in afterwards to continue providing contraception.

SEX AFTER THE MENOPAUSE

After the menopause there is no need to worry about becoming pregnant, and for many women this brings a feeling of liberation and greater enjoyment to sex. And many women do have wonderful sex lives after their periods finish. However, there are two problems that can, and often do, rear their heads in the years following the change – vaginal dryness and lack of libido.

Both are due to the very low levels of oestrogen that inevitably happens when the ovaries stop working.

Bethany, age 56

'My husband was quite a bit older than me, and died when I was only 51. To begin with, having a new relationship was the last thing on my mind – apart from missing him dreadfully, I had to support our kids, who were at college. But after a few years, I did meet someone new, who I really liked. But when it came to having sex, I just couldn't get aroused. I stayed as dry as a bone – and it was uncomfortable for both of us. I was embarrassed, and thought he would think I didn't fancy him, which wasn't true. There was no way I could discuss it with my doctor, but one evening, after I'd had a couple of glasses of wine, I mentioned it to a girlfriend. She told me the same thing had happened to her, and that she used a lubricant designed for older women. I didn't find it easy to go shopping for it – silly really – but now I have a supply it does really help, and I've managed to tell my partner that its nothing to do with him, it's just that I've lost my oestrogen.'

Vaginal dryness

Oestrogen has a moisture-retaining effect on the skin, and this means that after the menopause the skin does become noticeably drier and thinner – not only in the more obvious places, like your face, but also in the not-so-obvious, particularly the genital area. It's a condition known medically as atrophic vaginitis. Many women just notice that sex is dry and uncomfortable, no matter how much foreplay you have, and the lubricating glands that help make sex enjoyable just don't work any more. Other symptoms include the vulva feeling a bit itchy and sore, and this is often mistaken for thrush. Sometimes the dryness is so extreme that it leads to inflammation, which can cause slight bleeding or a vaginal discharge. A dry, inflamed vulva and vagina is also at increased risk from infection from organisms from around the anus. The change in the genital tissues can also increase the risk of urinary problems, particularly urinary tract infections.

Tests and treatment

If you look at your vulva yourself, using a mirror, you may be able to see that the tissues around the entrance to the vagina look much paler than they used to when you were younger. But don't try to make a diagnosis yourself – if you have an uncomfortable vulva or vagina, or are finding sex uncomfortable, go and see your GP. A good doctor will be able to make the diagnosis straight away, from the characteristic appearance of the genital tissues, but if you have been having itching or a discharge as well, swabs should be taken to rule out an infection. Occasionally other problems can be to blame, particularly lichen sclerosus (see page 233) and any woman who has vaginal bleeding after the menopause should have a pelvic scan to rule out causes other than simple inflammation.

Lubricating agents

A number of lubricating agents available from chemists and supermarkets can give relief from vaginal dryness. They can certainly make intercourse much more enjoyable, and improve day-to-day comfort. Bio-adhesive products, such as Replens, Senselle and Balance Activ Menopause Moisture Gel, aim to replace moisture in cells and are generally more effective, and longer lasting, than water-based gels such as KY jelly, which is more slippery.

HRT

The most effective way of dealing with atrophic vaginitis is to boost oestrogen levels again. One way to do this is with HRT (see page 59). This has the added advantage of often helping out with a flagging libido as well – which I'll deal with a bit later in this chapter. However, the risks associated with taking HRT (especially stroke and breast cancer) mean that in general it's not recommended for treating just atrophic vaginitis. That doesn't mean you can't use it if you want to – it should be a matter of personal choice. And HRT can be a very good treatment option if you have other problems as well, such as hot flushes or thinning bones.

Topical oestrogen

The other way of boosting oestrogen levels is to apply the hormone just where it's needed, in the vulva and vaginal area. This can be done via pessaries, creams or a ring. Several different brands are available, and in general pessaries inserted into the vagina are much less messy than creams. All types work, and can make the whole vulval area more moist and comfortable, and make sex enjoyable again – though you may still need to use a little extra lubricant. Topical oestrogens can also help prevent a problem with recurrent urinary infections.

Like other types of hormone replacement, topical oestrogens only work as long as you use them – once you stop using them, the symptoms will, unfortunately, tend to recur. The usual practice is to use your preferred treatment daily to begin with, to 're-oestrogenise' the area, then use a maintenance dose a couple of times a week. How long you use this type of treatment depends very much on personal circumstances – some women need a couple of courses a year, others need to use it most of the time.

The ring, Estring, is placed in the vagina and slowly releases estradiol over a period of three months, when it can then be replaced. It is only licensed for use for up to two years.

How long can topical treatments be used?

Very little of the oestrogen from these treatments is absorbed into the bloodstream, and there is no evidence that they can increase the risk of breast cancer or DVT. All women using them should be warned that the information leaflet inside the packaging has data based on the use of oestrogens taken by mouth, which is not accurate for topically used oestrogen. However, there is a slight question mark about whether oestrogens used in the genital area can cause a build-up in the lining of the womb. In the past, it was common practice to give a two-week course of oral progestogen once every six months to women using topical oestrogens regularly. Any bleeding at the end of the course of progesterone indicates that there had been some endometrial stimulation. This rule still applies to those using cream containing conjugated equine oestrogen and estriol, but absorption is much less from pessaries containing estradiol. It's not known exactly how long topical oestrogen can safely be used – no research has been done. The general guidelines are to use the lowest possible dose to relieve symptoms, and to use a product based on estradiol. The most popular in use in the UK is estradiol 10mcg pessaries. Current guidelines are that as long as a very low dose (10mcg estradiol pessaries) are used, then there is no need to use any additional Progestogen to protect the womb lining. However, any vaginal bleeding, even if it's only a couple of spots, should be reported to your doctor.

Be kind to your skin

The drier skin that occurs after the menopause is also much more prone to irritation from other chemicals, such as perfumes in bath products and shower gels, and enzymes in biological washing powders, and also just slightly uncomfortable underwear. Lace on knickers, and even wearing a panty liner, may trigger some irritation. Applying a (plain, unperfumed) moisturising cream to the genital area each day can help, but as always prevention is better than a cure, and plain cotton 'big knickers', washed in non-biological detergent with no fabric conditioner, can be a godsend for everyday use.

Bleeding after sex

The dryness and inflammation that can affect the vagina after the menopause can occasionally lead to slight bleeding after sex. But this should never be heavy – just slight spotting. And even though the cause may be obvious, it's still important to have any vaginal bleeding that occurs after the menopause checked out by a doctor. Occasionally it's due to a polyp, or, worse, it can be a sign of cancer. So don't ignore it.

Lichen sclerosus

This is a skin condition that can affect the vulva at any age, including childhood, but is more common in older women. It is thought to be an autoimmune condition, where the skin is attacked by the body's own immune system, and this leads to inflammation, which in turn leads to soreness and itching. It causes discomfort when passing urine, and can make sex very painful. Left untreated, the inflamed skin can become scarred, the normal structure of the skin of the vulva is lost and the inner labia may become fused together. Initially it is often mistaken for thrush, and many women only go and see their GP after months of suffering and finding that thrush treatments bought from the chemist don't help at all.

A GP with a knowledge of the condition can usually spot it immediately, as the skin looks white and scarred, but it's usual for a biopsy to be taken to confirm the diagnosis. Treatment is with a high-strength steroid cream, which needs to be used every day until the inflammation settles, which usually takes about three months.

Lichen sclerosus is a long-term condition which tends to flare up from time to time, and intermittent use of steroids for many years is usually required. This is important, as the condition can, very slightly, increase the risk of vulval cancer. However, this risk is vastly reduced if the inflammation is kept under control.

Sexually transmitted infections

Just because you are no longer at risk of becoming pregnant does not mean that having sex is risk-free – older women are just as vulnerable to contracting sexually transmitted infections as younger women if they have sex with an infected partner. Changing sexual practice, with more older women having new relationships after the breakdown of a long-term relationship, has meant that the rate of diagnosis of all sexually transmitted infections, but particularly chlamydia, has been on the rise in women over 40 in the UK.

So even if you no longer need contraception, it is important to take the same precautions as younger, fertile women when having sex. If you are with a new partner, use condoms (a cap is another option, but not quite as good) until you have both had full STI testing and are sure you are in a monogamous relationship. The best place to get tests done is a genito-urinary medicine clinic, but if the thought of that freaks you out, see your GP or practice nurse. Remember, everything in the consulting room is confidential, so it is safe to be honest, and that way you will get the right tests done.

Libido and the menopause

Abigail, age 60

'My husband and I had always had sex at least twice a week.
It had always been an important and enjoyable part of our
relationship. After the menopause, to begin with I enjoyed sex
even more, as I wasn't worrying about getting pregnant. But
then I realised I didn't really feel like having sex any more – I
just wanted to get to sleep. To begin with my husband didn't say
anything, but when he asked me if I was having an affair I knew
I had to do something. I told him it was nothing to do with him –
that it was me – though I knew he found it difficult. He thought
I'd gone off him, which wasn't true. I still found him attractive, I
just didn't seem to want sex any more.

My GP was sympathetic, but it was clear there was no real
answer. I wasn't keen on taking HRT, as my periods had stopped
three years previously, and I was over my flushes and sweats.
And I knew my husband wouldn't want me to increase my risk
of breast cancer just for the sake of our sex life. Interestingly,
talking about the problem honestly with my husband really
helped, and actually my sex drive has come back a bit. I know it
will never be the same as it was when I was younger – but then,
my husband doesn't find getting an erection as easy as he did.
We just have to accept that this is part of the change that comes
with getting a bit older.'

Libido is a complex subject that is controlled by many different
factors, including the state of your relationship, general physical and
mental health, as well as hormones. So not surprisingly there is no
general rule about what happens at the menopause.

Some women find the freedom from worrying about an unwanted

pregnancy or having to bother about contraception a real boost to their sex drive, and find their libido surges when their periods stop.

However, unfortunately a more common scenario is for women to notice that their libido diminishes in the years that follow the menopause. They simply don't feel like having sex any more, and when they do, they don't find it so enjoyable. It takes longer to become aroused, and the genital area becomes less sensitive to touching and stroking.

The reason for this, yet again, is the fall in hormones that occurs when the ovaries stop functioning. And this time it's not just low oestrogen levels that are to blame, but testosterone as well.

Testosterone? In women?

The ovaries produce testosterone from puberty onwards, but unlike oestrogen, the amount produced declines slowly from the twenties onwards, so by the time you reach the menopause the levels are only about half those produced in the twenties.

The testosterone produced by the ovaries has an important role in sex drive, and also to a lesser extent in the structure of bones and muscles, skin and hair. Even in women, who produce only tiny quantities compared to men, it's an important hormone.

A small amount of testosterone is also produced by the adrenal glands, and after the menopause, when oestrogen levels fall, it becomes the dominant influence on hair, but it's not enough to boost sex drive. The best studies on the influence of testosterone on libido have been done on women who have had their ovaries removed, pre-menopause, who are therefore plunged into an immediate 'surgical' menopause. Many of these women report a drop in their sex drive, and in clinical trials those given testosterone supplements have been shown to have a significant improvement in libido compared to those given placebo. For this reason, testosterone has been promoted as a treatment for low libido in post-menopausal women, and some studies have indicated that it can improve not only sex drive, but also mood and a general sense of wellbeing.

However, testosterone can cause side effects, such as greasy skin, acne, excess facial hair, and also increase the tendency to make pattern hair loss on the scalp. It can also cause changes in liver function, though this is rare. For this reason it is usually only given when its masculinising effects can be counterbalanced by oestrogen. In other words, if you're going to use testosterone, it's best to have HRT as well, and the combination can be really good for a lot of women, though of course, it's not side-effect-free.

Can I get replacement testosterone?

In the past, testosterone was available for women in the form of a skin patch, but this has now been withdrawn. Currently, the only licensed form of testosterone for women in the UK is an implant which is placed under the skin, and releases testosterone for six months. If it causes unwanted side effects there is nothing you can do about it – the implant is so small it's impossible to remove, and for this reason it's not a popular option. Another option is Tibolone, a unique form of HRT that has oestrogenic, progestogenic and also a testosterone-like action, all in one daily pill. The oestrogen-like dose (it's a synthetic oestrogen) is quite high, and side effects can be more troublesome, therefore it's not generally used as a first-line option for women wanting treatment for hot flushes. And opting to improve your sex life at the risk of increasing your chance of breast cancer and blood clots is not every woman's choice. That said, it can be a good choice if you are having awful flushes and problems with a lowered sex drive.

Probably the best way of getting testosterone is by using a small amount of the gel that is designed for men requiring testosterone replacement therapy. It's not licensed for women, and therefore many doctors, including specialists, won't prescribe it. Not only that, but the dose women require is unknown – the concentration in the 'male' gel is considerably higher than that in the gel intended for women.

I have prescribed it, advising women to use only a tiny amount each day, and have done regular blood tests of their testosterone to check that they have not accidentally been using too much.

So that's the theory, but how does it work in practice? Here are some real-life case histories.

Rachel, age 49

HER STORY: I've been on the Pill nearly all my life – apart from when I had the kids, and it's suited me really well. Now I'm 49 I'm wondering if I should stop. I'm not having any menopausal symptoms, but surely at my age I don't need contraception, even though my periods are still as regular as clockwork each month?

MORE BACKGROUND INFORMATION: Rachel was taking the combined pill, containing both oestrogen and progesterone. She was fit and healthy, had an active lifestyle, was not overweight and had never smoked, so the combined pill was a good option for her, even in her late forties. However, the hormones it contained were responsible for her regular periods and also would be giving her plenty of oestrogen, completely masking what was going on in her own ovaries. As long as she was taking it she would have no menopausal symptoms.

MY ADVICE: The only way to know if she was menopausal or not would be for her to stop the Pill. However, I warned her that she should not assume she could not get pregnant – it could be that her ovaries had several more years of life in them, so I advised her that it was important she used some form of contraception until it was clear what was happening in her body. A barrier method would be best in the short term.

If her cycle resumed a regular pattern off the Pill, she could consider having a coil – either a copper one or, better still, a Mirena, as this would provide more long-term contraception without interfering with the functioning of her ovaries. However, there was also a possibility that her ovaries had already run out of follicles, and when she stopped the Pill she would be plunged into an immediate menopause, and the very sudden fall in her oestrogen levels would lead to hot flushes and sweats.

She stopped the Pill, and though her periods did return, they were very erratic, and she started having a few flushes and sweats, so it was clear she was in the perimenopause. I advised her that if the flushes got worse, she was a good candidate for HRT, but she said she wanted to leave her body free of hormones for a while.

Nadia, age 53

HER STORY: I've been dating a new partner for a couple of weeks, and last week we had sex. Stupidly, I didn't ask him to use a condom. It just didn't cross my mind, as my periods stopped three years ago. But now I've got a discharge, and I'm sore, and I'm really worried I've got some nasty infection.

MORE BACKGROUND INFORMATION: Nadia had been single since her divorce in her mid-forties and she'd had 'quite a few' partners. She had asked them to use condoms while she was still having periods, but since the menopause she hadn't bothered, as she was no longer concerned about an unwanted pregnancy. She herself admitted that this had been risky, and that she was lucky that she hadn't run into trouble with an infection before.

MY ADVICE: Swab tests confirmed that she had chlamydia. Not only did she need antibiotics, but she also needed to tell her new partner about her infection. I also advised her that she ought to have blood tests done to check for HIV, and though I could do this at the surgery, she would get a quicker result if she went to a genito-urinary clinic. I warned her that it would take four weeks for the test to show HIV acquired from her recent contact, so she would need another repeat test done then.

Camilla, age 56

HER STORY: My vagina feels dry and a bit itchy, it's uncomfortable to have sex and I feel really sore afterwards. I've tried using KY jelly, but it hasn't really helped. I don't have any discharge, but I'm wondering if I've got thrush?

MORE BACKGROUND INFORMATION: Camilla had gone through the menopause at 51, and though she'd had a few flushes and dizzy spells, it hadn't bothered her that much, and she was delighted not to have to cope with periods any more. She'd been married for 30 years, and though she said her sex drive had dropped a bit, she felt this was normal for such a long relationship and she still had sex a couple of times a month.

MY ADVICE: On examination, Camilla had the classic changes of atrophic vaginitis. Her genital tissues looked paler than in the pre-menopausal woman, and the lining of her vagina looked slightly inflamed. Swabs confirmed that she did not have an infection.

I advised that she use topical oestrogen, in the form of pessaries, to plump up her genital tissues. This would also improve her sexual response during sex, but I also suggested she switch the KY jelly for an oil-based lubricant.

A month later she reported a great improvement. I suggested she continue using the pessaries twice a week for three months, then she could stop them and see how things went. If she became dry again, which was likely, she could start using them once more.

Felicity, age 55

HER STORY: I just don't feel like having sex any more. I've been with my second husband 10 years now, and we used to have a great sex life. I still love him, but I just can't think why I ever bothered with sex. It honestly wouldn't bother me if I never had sex again, but obviously it would bother my husband, so I need to do something about it. Would HRT help?

MORE BACKGROUND INFORMATION: Felicity went through the menopause at 49, and she'd been able to cope with the flushes and sweats that she'd initially had, and now they had gone. She admitted her vagina was dry during sex, but thought that this was because she wasn't aroused – she was only having sex to please her husband. She was a little overweight, but her blood pressure was normal and there was no family history of breast cancer. She did, though, like her wine, and admitted she probably drank a bit more than she should.

MY ADVICE: As her relationship was otherwise fine, it was likely that Felicity's lost libido was because of her lack of hormones. HRT would probably help her, but it came with the slightly increased risk of breast cancer, though she could help reduce her risk overall by cutting back on her wine intake. She wanted a simple regime, so I gave her tablets containing both oestrogen and progesterone to be taken each day. Initially she felt bloated, but her libido began to improve within weeks. She admitted it was not as good as before the menopause, so I suggested she could have some extra testosterone, using a tiny amount of the gel usually prescribed for men. I warned her that its use was not officially licensed in women, and that she would need regular checks of her liver function while she was using it. She decided not to bother for the time being – she said the gel sounded a bit of a faff, and she didn't want blood tests. However, she would bear it in mind for the future if her libido fell again.

SUMMARY

📖 Women should continue to use contraception until a year after their last period. Up until this time it's still possible to ovulate and have a surprise pregnancy.

📖 There is a wide choice of contraception suitable for women in their forties, including the combined pill, though this will mask any signs of the menopause.

📖 Women of all ages can, and do, get sexually transmitted infections. After the menopause you are no longer at risk of an unwanted pregnancy, but it's still very important to protect yourself against infections, especially when you are with a new partner.

📖 The fall in hormone levels, especially oestrogen and testosterone, can lead to a dramatic decline in libido after the menopause. This can be improved with HRT or testosterone replacement, but both of these carry other health risks.

📖 Another common problem after the menopause is vaginal dryness, again caused by low levels of oestrogen. This can lead to vaginal discomfort, especially during sex, and also occasionally some slight itching. It can easily be treated with oestrogen cream or pessaries, applied directly to the genital area.

📖 Most post-menopausal women need some form of artificial lubrication to make sex more comfortable. Oil-based products, such as Senselle, are generally much more effective for this than water-based ones, such as KY jelly.

9

WATERWORKS AND PELVIC FLOOR

There comes a time in most women's lives when you realise that your bladder and pelvic area isn't quite the same as it was when you were young. You've come to terms with the fact that your vagina couldn't possibly remain completely unchanged after having a baby (even though you thought at the time it would be), but then you realise that it's just not your tummy muscles that seem to have disappeared. Everything has moved south, and is bulging.

Having slackness in your pelvic area may not cause you any problems, but it can mean that you don't feel as much during sex, simply because your vagina is larger than it used to be before. Alternatively, if your womb has dropped a little, your vagina is shorter, so sex can be more uncomfortable.

Then there is the not-so-little issue of bladder problems. It's rare for a woman to go through life without at least one episode of 'urinary trouble' and most have considerably more than just the one. But the nature of the problems, and the symptoms they cause, change through the years, and the big problem for slightly older women, especially after the menopause, is incontinence.

I'm not talking here about the severe incontinence that affects the very elderly and infirm, who may have little, if any, control of their bladder. What I'm talking about is accidentally passing urine, sometimes just a tiny drop, sometimes a bit more, at any time.

Bladder weakness is incredibly common – a survey by the Royal College of Physicians revealed that 24 per cent of older people suffer from accidental leakage of urine, and it's thought that at least three million women in the UK are regularly incontinent. In the past it was barely mentioned, but adverts for pads on the TV and notices on the backs of the doors of public loos mean it is coming more into the public radar. But it still isn't discussed nearly as much as it should be and sadly many women suffer from it for years before seeking medical help, thinking that a 'little leakage' is a normal part of ageing. And that's a real shame, as it's a treatable problem that can often be completely cured.

As with the other chapters, I'll start with the questions I'm often asked in my surgery, then go on to more detailed background information, then finish up with some case histories.

I've noticed that I can't feel very much during sex. It changed a little bit after I had my kids, but since the menopause it's as if my vagina has gone all floppy and lost its tone. Is this normal?

Your vagina will have been stretched by childbirth, especially if you had big babies or had a forceps delivery. Oestrogen helps to maintain the tone of the genital tissues, and after this is lost at the menopause the tissues do tend to become thinner and more floppy, so pre-existing changes become more noticeable. You can help to tighten things up at the entrance to the vagina by doing pelvic-floor exercises, and this can make sex more enjoyable. (There is more information about these on page 252.) However, if it continues to be a problem, the only solution may be to have surgery to remove the excess vaginal lining, and also tighten up the tissues that support the vaginal wall. (See page 254 for more information.)

I can feel 'something coming down' in my vagina. Is this my womb? What can I do about it?

Yes, it's likely to be your womb. The ligaments that support the uterus become more slack with age, and this allows it to drop down a little into the vagina. It tends to occur more commonly in women who have had children. Unfortunately, you can't tone up these muscles with exercise, and if you are very uncomfortable, or sex is difficult, it's best corrected by surgery. There are a variety of different procedures available, so see page 266 for more information.

Sometimes the sensation of something coming down in the vagina is not from the womb but from the vaginal walls, either the front one – an anterior prolapse – or the back wall – a posterior prolapse (see page 261).

I seem to need to go the loo to pass urine far more than my friends. They all laugh that I know where all the public loos are in town, but I'd love to be able to go out and not worry about being near a toilet.

Occasionally this is caused by a urine infection, so you should get this checked by your GP. However, more commonly it's just a result of always going to the toilet frequently (which may have started in childhood) so your bladder has got used to never being stretched very much. This type of problem often gets worse after the menopause, when the genital tissues become generally thinner. You can train your bladder to hold more by hanging on and trying not to go so often. It can help to keep a diary of how often you go, to track your progress. There is more information about this on page 257.

I've started to leak a bit of urine when I do exercise, such as jogging or playing tennis. I now daren't go out to do any sport without wearing a pad. Why is this, and what can I do about it?

This is what is known as stress incontinence. It's due to lack of support at the bottom of the bladder, which sags downwards at the opening of the outlet valve. This tends to happen when the pressure in the abdominal cavity increases, such as when you are doing sport and also when you cough or sneeze. The lack of support for the bladder is usually caused by sagging of the front vaginal wall. The original damage often occurs in childbirth, but it's often after the menopause that symptoms appear, as the tissues become generally more slack when oestrogen levels fall. Pelvic-floor exercises can often make a huge difference, as long as you do them often enough (see page 252) but if leaking continues a variety of surgical techniques are available. (See page 254 for more information on this.)

I often suddenly need to pass urine and find it difficult to hang on. I've recently had a few accidents, which is really embarrassing – it just happens out of the blue. Why is this?

This is what's known as 'urge incontinence'. It's caused by the muscles in the bladder wall suddenly going into spasm, often when the bladder only contains a small amount of urine. It can usually be successfully treated with tablets that relax the bladder muscle, though side effects of these, such as a dry mouth and constipation, can be a problem.

My bladder is very unreliable – I often have to dash to the loo and sometimes I barely make it. I've also had some leaking when I've run for the bus. I've resorted to wearing panty liners, but I find they make my skin quite sore, especially at the back on my buttocks. They also sometimes don't cope with the leaking. There is no way I want those big, bulky incontinence pads, but what would you suggest?

This sounds like 'mixed incontinence' – a combination of stress and urge incontinence. It may be due to an infection, so get this checked by your GP. If not, there are treatments available for this, and with mixed incontinence you may be offered a combination of both tablets, and maybe surgery, but beforehand it would best to have tests done on your bladder – a 'urodynamic assessment' (see page 249). If you do have to resort to pads (and I hope after reading this that you won't, or at least only short term while you are waiting for treatment), those specifically designed for the purpose, such as Tena, are far better than sanitary towels. They have better absorbency where it's needed and are less likely to cause skin irritation or rashes.

INCONTINENCE

There are two main types of incontinence in women – stress incontinence and urge incontinence. It's important to sort out which type you have, as their treatments are very different. Some women have just one type, others a mix of both. Another problem that can occur is frequency – which is needing to go to the loo very often, more than eight times a day, every day. This may occur on its own, or together with incontinence.

The bladder is a bit like a balloon, with a thin, delicate, inner lining that is surrounded by a wall of muscles. It expands as it fills with urine, and the outlet – the urethra – has a sphincter which is normally closed until you voluntarily decide to open it. The action of the sphincter is helped by the muscles beneath the bladder that surround and support the urethra – the pelvic floor muscles.

The amount of urine that the bladder can hold before it feels full varies between individuals, but is usually around 300 to 400ml. Complex messages pass between the bladder, the pelvic-floor muscles and the brain. These tell you when your bladder feels full and also allow you to contract the bladder muscles and relax the pelvic-floor muscles so it can be emptied.

Urodynamic tests

Sometimes it's easy to sort out which type of problem you have just from your symptoms, but if you are not sure, urodynamic investigations can help. These are done in a specialist hospital clinic (usually a urogynaecology clinic) and involve drinking a large amount of water and having the pressure inside your bladder monitored as it fills. The test will also monitor how much urine your bladder is holding when you feel the need to go to the loo, and when you start passing urine. It's not painful in any way, but I know some women find it embarrassing. However, it's far less embarrassing than continuing to leak urine.

Stress incontinence

Elizabeth, age 47

'The first time it happened I was running for the bus on the way to work. I realised I'd leaked a bit of urine, and even though I was wearing dark clothing, I was worried that someone would be able to smell me. I also hated the feeling of my damp underwear. After it happened again the following week I took to wearing panty liners, but after wearing them every day for three months my skin felt a bit sore. I only ever leaked when I was doing something active, but as I was only 45 I wanted to do something about it. I was too young to be wearing pads all the time. My doctor told me I had stress incontinence, and that my pelvic-floor muscles were weak. No one had mentioned pelvic-floor exercises to me after I'd had my children, or if they had, I didn't take it in. Anyway, she gave me an instruction sheet on how to do them. I wasn't sure I was doing the right thing, so a friend suggested some special weighted vaginal cones. To begin with they just fell out, but gradually I got my pelvic floor stronger and I can now keep a light cone in place. The 'accidents' have now got much less, so for now I'm just going to keep on with the exercises, but I'm aware I may need some sort of surgery if it gets worse when I'm older.'

Stress incontinence is the accidental leaking of urine that occurs when you cough, sneeze, run, or just even laugh. It's the most common type of incontinence in women, and as many as one in five women over 40 have some degree of stress incontinence, though it's likely that the true number is much higher than this, as many women suffer from it but never report it to their doctor.

Why me?

Most cases of stress incontinence are due to weakened pelvic-floor muscles, and the damage is done during childbirth. Both pregnancy and especially a vaginal delivery can put an enormous strain on the pelvic-floor muscles. The more babies you have, and the bigger they are, the greater the chance of stretching and weakening these all-important muscles. Many women notice they are slightly incontinent in the weeks after giving birth, but the problem often gets better even with only half-hearted pelvic-floor exercises. But after the menopause the tissues of the genital area all change, the muscles become weaker still and the problem rears its head again, only this time it's much worse. Stress incontinence is also more common in those who are overweight (the pelvic muscles are simply under more strain, all the time) and in those who have a chronic smokers' cough.

Do I need any tests?

Having a urine infection always makes bladder problems worse, and in older women an infection may not cause the classic burning and stinging that you get when you have cystitis as a young woman. So all women with bladder problems should have a urine sample tested for bacteria.

Though stress incontinence can usually be diagnosed from the symptoms alone, if there is any question about whether there may be mixed incontinence, urodymanic tests can be helpful in establishing an exact diagnosis.

What can be done about it?

Treatment first and foremost is 'self-help'. Losing weight and stopping smoking can help, but the most important action to take is to strengthen the pelvic-floor muscles. About 60 per cent of cases of stress incontinence can be cured, or nearly cured, with this alone.

As with any other muscles, the more you exercise them the stronger they will become. And it's never too late to start – even if the damage was done 20, 30 years ago, when your offspring were born, you can still do a great deal of repair work yourself.

Pelvic-floor exercises

First, a word of caution. Toning up your pelvic floor is not easy. Neither is it something that can be done overnight. As with other muscles, to make a difference you have to work the muscles regularly, certainly at least once a day (and preferably more than this) for at least three months. If you want your intimate parts to stay toned, you have to do some maintenance work as well.

But all this hard work can pay dividends, putting an end to stress incontinence and improving your sex life as well.

First you need to identify the right muscles, and this is easier said than done. The best way to do this is to try stopping the urine flow when you are peeing. Hold for a slow count of three, then relax, and start peeing again. Do this until you feel you really have good control of the flow, repeatedly stopping and starting again. I should emphasise that this exercise should be done merely so that you know where the muscles are, as many experts feel that stopping the flow of urine repeatedly over a long period of time is not a good idea and could lead to urinary tract infections. So once you know where the muscles are, switch to tightening and relaxing the muscles at other times – when you are sitting watching TV, doing the ironing, or even while waiting at traffic lights. Repeat as often as possible – aim for at least 30 contractions a day.

The next step is to work on the muscles a little further back, around the vagina and anus. Squeeze as if you are holding first a tampon, then as if you are trying to stop yourself passing wind. Again, hold and repeat.

If you are finding it really hard to identify the right muscles, seeing a specialist physiotherapist can be very helpful. Alternatively, there are various devices that are available that can help you 'train' your pelvic-floor muscles. I personally recommend devices that are placed in the vagina and give an electrical impulse to tighten the muscles, such as the Pelviva system. Weighted cones are often mentioned, but don't even try to use these unless you have done some preliminary exercises first, otherwise it's just too depressing. They just fall out.

What if exercises don't work? What other treatment is available?

The main treatment for persistent stress incontinence is some sort of surgical technique to hitch up the bladder neck, or to tighten the structures below the base of the bladder.

What about pills?

The drug duloxetine is a relatively new medical treatment for stress incontinence. It is thought to work by increasing the activity of the nerve that stimulates the sphincter. It's not suitable for everyone, though (including smokers as well as people who have had heart problems or certain types of mental health conditions), and it frequently causes side effects, such as a dry mouth, constipation, nausea and tiredness. However, it is worth a try, especially if you are keen to avoid surgery.

Surgical methods - what is available?

There are various different types of operation, and which one is used depends on individual circumstances.

Tapes

If you just have weakness around the entrance to the bladder, placing a supporting tape around it may be all that is required, which is known as a tension-free vaginal tape procedure. It can be done under either local or general anaesthetic; the tape is inserted through a small cut in the front vaginal wall, then threaded through two small holes on the lower abdominal wall just below the pubic bone, forming a loop around the urethra. Long-term success rates are still being evaluated, but five-year success rates are between 72 and 84 per cent.

The operation is only suitable for women who have completed their families and who do not have significant prolapse.

A similar procedure is Transobturator Tape (TOT). This is inserted through three small cuts: one in the vagina and one on each side of the upper inner thigh. This operation is often done when there is both stress and urge incontinence.

Colposuspension

This is a more major operation that is performed under general anaesthetic. It involves opening up the lower abdominal wall and lifting up the base of the bladder by stitching the lower part of the front of the vagina to a ligament behind the pubic bone. It used to be the most commonly performed operation, but has largely now been replaced with less invasive surgery. The operation can be done via keyhole surgery, but success rates with this method are generally not as good as with open surgery. Success rates overall are between 50 and 70 per cent.

As with all operations there are risks to both Tension-free Vaginal Tape (TVT) and colposuspension procedures, such as bleeding, pain and infection, though the overall risk of these is low. The most common problem is difficulty in passing urine afterwards (in other words, going from one extreme to the other) and a catheter may be needed for a few days. A few women may find they have difficulty completely emptying their bladder afterwards, which can increase the risk of urinary infections.

'Repair' surgery

Stress incontinence can also occur if the lower part of the bladder bulges into the vagina (known medically as a cystocele) or if the urethra bulges into the vagina (a urethrocele). Unfortunately, although pelvic floor exercises can tighten up the muscles that support the bladder, they can't tighten up the vaginal wall. It may also be linked to prolapse of the womb itself, and for these conditions 'repair surgery' may be required. This is discussed in the section on page 266.

Urge incontinence

Emilia, age 60

'I'd always had to go to the loo fairly frequently, but since the menopause it's got a bit worse. I find myself having to dash to the toilet suddenly, and on a few occasions I've started wetting myself before I've got there. Awful. I started wearing sanitary towels again, but even so I got panicky if I had to sit in the middle of a row at the cinema where I couldn't get out easily, or if I was anywhere where I didn't know where there was a toilet. I dreaded weddings. I'd avoid having anything to drink for hours before we went anywhere if I thought I wouldn't have easy access to a toilet. My whole life was being ruled by my unreliable bladder. I plucked up courage to mention it to the lovely nurse at the surgery when I went for my smear test, and she immediately booked me in to see one of the doctors who specialised in women's problems. She checked that I didn't have a urine infection, and told me I had an unstable bladder. She gave me tablets, which helped a bit, but gave me an awful dry mouth, so I only took them when I knew I was going out. So she then arranged for me to see a specialist, and I had some more tests on my bladder, which involved peeing when someone measured the pressure in my bladder. But I didn't mind – I just wanted the problem sorted. It turns out that not only is my bladder muscle overactive, but that my bladder is very small, probably a result of all those years of going to the loo so frequently. So now I'm training myself not to go so often, which isn't easy, but it is working. I even managed to get through my son's three-hour graduation ceremony without worrying about needing to go to the toilet.'

Urge incontinence is when you have a sudden uncontrollable urge to pass urine, and holding on until you get to the loo is nigh on impossible. Affected women get very little warning that they need to pass urine (known medically as 'urgency') and may have to urinate very frequently, sometimes as often as every half an hour.

Normally, the bladder fills very slowly and the muscles in its walls send a signal to the brain, in good time, to tell you that it's full. But in some people the muscles contract at the wrong time, often when there is very little urine inside the bladder. It's called an overactive bladder, and at its worst it can lead to urge incontinence – the muscles contract so much that the bladder empties, no matter how hard you try to stop it happening.

How often a 'normal' person empties their bladder depends a lot on how much they drink, and also on the weather – if it's hot you lose a lot of water through sweat and don't need to go to the loo so often. On the other hand, if you drink ten mugs of coffee or tea each day you are bound to be a frequent visitor to the girl's room. But as a general rule, it's normal to go to the loo to empty your bladder up to eight times a day, and once or twice at night. If you are consistently going more than this, you may have an overactive bladder.

Why me?

It can occur at any age but is especially common in post-menopausal women. Often there is no obvious cause, but lack of oestrogen plays a part, and being overweight makes it worse, as this puts extra pressure on the bladder.

Do I need any tests?

Sometimes the symptoms of an overactive bladder can be due to a urinary tract infection (UTI), and in older women this may be the only symptom – there may not be the pain that classically goes with cystitis in younger women. So it's always worth taking a sample to your GP for analysis, as all you may need is a course of antibiotics to sort the problem.

What can be done about it?

Unlike stress incontinence, urge incontinence is not treated with surgery (unless you have stress incontinence as well). Instead, bladder retraining and drugs are used.

Self-help

There is quite a lot you can do to help yourself to stop passing urine quite so often. Top of the list is to lose weight, and also to cut down on caffeine and alcohol, as these irritate the lining of the bladder. The stronger they are, the worse the effect, so if you need that morning boost, get it from a cup of instant, not a double espresso – especially if you know you've got to sit on a bus or train with no loo to get to work. And from what my patients tell me, gin is notoriously bad news for irritable bladders.

However, it's not a good idea to cut down on the amount of fluid you drink, which is what many women do, as this can make your urine very concentrated, which in itself can irritate the bladder and urethra and increase the risk of a bladder infection. Aim to drink around two litres of fluid a day, more if the weather is hot.

Bladder retraining

This, as its name suggests, trains your bladder to hold more urine. Your bladder is like your stomach – it gets used to holding a certain volume, and in the same way that people who eat small meals have a small stomach, the more often you go to the loo, the more often you'll need to go. So what you need to do is learn to suppress or somehow try to ignore the need to pee. That way the bladder gradually gets used to holding more urine, and eventually you won't feel the need to go so often. This means 'holding on' when you feel the need to pee, and also avoiding going 'just in case' unless it's really necessary. To do this well you need to keep a diary of how often you are going, and ideally measure how much urine you pass each time. Sounds a bit yucky, I know, but remember urine is sterile. Just keep a cheap plastic measuring jug in the loo for the purpose, and rinse it out afterwards. Eventually you should be able to throw it away, as it won't be needed any more. Chart your progress week by week – it can be very satisfying seeing your bladder capacity increase. It can also help to set yourself some targets. Aim initially to hold on for an extra 10 minutes, then gradually work up to half an hour, and so on. If you are worried about having an accident, wear a panty liner. If you find you can't do this on your own, a specialist continence nurse can help with bladder re-training – ask your GP for a referral.

Medical treatments

There are a number of different drugs that can help with an overactive bladder and urge incontinence, such as oxybutynin, tolterodine and solifenacin. They all work by relaxing the muscles of the bladder, but side effects such as a dry mouth and constipation are quite common. Generally, the higher the dose, the worse the side effects are likely to be, so I always recommend starting with a low dose and increasing it until you have the right balance between the positive effect on the bladder and unwanted side effects. Side effects vary from person to person, and different drugs suit different people, so if one doesn't suit, it's worth trying another. Some are available as slow-release pills, while others can be given via skin patches, so it's also worth trying different delivery methods. Don't worry if you have to go back to your doctor several times, it's worth it to get the medicine that suits you best.

Botox

Botulinum toxin (Botox) is a powerful neurotoxin which blocks the message from the nerves that tells the muscles to contract. This means that injecting Botox into the bladder muscle can treat an overactive bladder and urge incontinence. The procedure is done under either local or general anaesthetic, and involves a telescope being passed into the bladder, then 20 or so small injections are given in different places throughout the bladder wall. The effects usually last about nine to 12 months, after which it can be repeated. It's usually successful in 70 to 80 per cent of patients, but it can lead to difficulties in passing urine and emptying the bladder in up to 20 per cent of cases. It is important to be fully counselled before undergoing Botox, so you are well aware of the risks in your particular case.

URINARY TRACT INFECTIONS

It's rare for a woman to go through life without getting at least one urinary tract infection. Basic anatomy is to blame, the urethra – the passage that takes urine from the bladder to the outside – is very short in women compared to men, and its orifice is close to the anus. That means it's incredibly easy for the bacteria in stools to accidentally spread to the genital area, and around the entrance to the urethra.

Cystitis, the medical term for inflammation of the bladder, tends to cause dramatic symptoms in younger women – a desperate need to pass urine, and when you do go, only a dribble comes out, and it feels as if you are peeing shards of glass. It's often linked to an increase in sexual activity, hence the term 'honeymoon cystitis', as the mechanics of intercourse push bugs up from the vulva into the bladder.

Women in their thirties and forties tend not to get urinary infections so often, but once you are past the menopause, things change again.

Why me?

Lack of oestrogen causes a change in the genital tissues, which become more dry and fragile. There is also a reduction in the naturally protective secretions, and this increases the risk of urinary tract infections occurring. As with younger women, urinary tract infections can be linked with sexual activity, but often there is no obvious reason for one to occur.

Symptoms and tests

Though there may be classic pain and stinging, symptoms of a urinary infection in older women may be much more subtle. Some just notice they need to pass water a bit more often and that their urine smells slightly strange. I have often treated women who have had symptoms of an infection for months before coming to my surgery – they just thought their increased visits to the loo were part of normal ageing.

Though symptoms are often the giveaway to the diagnosis, it's important to have an infection confirmed by analysis of a sample of urine in the laboratory, as frequency can just be a sign of an irritable bladder. Analysis is helpful in indicating which antibiotic needs to be used, as many of the causative bacteria are resistant to the commonly used treatments.

Prevention

No matter what your age, there are steps you can take to help prevent urinary infections, and the change in the tissues after the menopause means that all women should follow these basic rules.

- Always wipe front to back after you've been to the loo, especially after you have opened your bowels, never the other way round – it just drags bugs from around the anus towards the urethral entrance.

- Never douche or spray the shower head upwards around your vaginal area. It can force bacteria up into the bladder, and it's not good for vaginal health either – it washes away what few protective secretions you still have.

- Avoid using bubble baths and perfumed gels and soaps around the vulval area, especially if you have sensitive skin. Any inflammation in the skin makes it more prone to infection.

- Make sure your vagina is well lubricated during sex to avoid excess friction (which in turn will cause inflammation). After the menopause this usually means using extra lubricant from a tube or bottle – nature is not good at providing enough.

Treatment

Straightforward infections can be treated with antibiotics, which usually only need to be taken for three days. More steps are required if infections become a recurrent nuisance. Using topical oestrogen (as either pessaries or cream) around the vulva area (see page 231) can help improve the natural defences and can be really helpful in preventing recurrent attacks. Most women need an initial three-month course to plump up the cells again, and then need intermittent courses if infection recurs. Some women need to use topical oestrogen for years in order to prevent infections. This is safe as long as steps are taken to ensure the lining of the womb does not become thickened, which usually involves taking occasional courses of oral progesterone.

If infections continue despite topical oestrogen, it may be necessary to take a long course of low-dose antibiotics, usually for about three months, as a preventative measure.

PROLAPSE PROBLEMS

Maya, age 39

'I was realistic and knew that after I'd had my children my vagina would never be quite the same. It wasn't too bad after baby number one, but after the second, it definitely felt very different. Both my babies had been big – nearly 9lb each, so I knew everything had stretched, a lot. My vagina felt slack, and I couldn't feel much during sex, so I started going to Pilates classes and tried to work on my pelvic floor, but it didn't help. My vagina felt odd and bulgy, and sometimes I had difficulty passing a motion, even though my stools weren't hard. My doctor said my womb had dropped slightly, but the main problem was the back wall of my vagina, which was very slack. She recommended I see a gynaecologist, who recommended surgery. I didn't need to have my womb removed, just the back wall of my vagina tightened up. It was done as a day case at the local hospital, and though I was sore for a week afterwards, overall it wasn't too bad, and it was definitely worth having done. I feel much more comfortable now.'

The organs of the pelvis, including the bladder, lower large bowel and the womb, are normally firmly held in place not only by the pelvic-floor muscles but also by strong ligaments which pass to the bones of the pelvis. If these ligaments are weakened, the organs move with gravity downwards, and the space available for them to do this is the vagina. The result is what is known as a prolapse.

There are different types of prolapse depending on which organ has dropped, and also differing degrees of prolapse. Sometimes the womb, or the bowel, only shifts a little, and causes no symptoms, but a larger prolapse can result in part of the wall of the vagina or, worse still, the cervix, dropping right through the vagina so it can be felt on the outside.

Having some degree of a prolapse is incredibly common. Exact statistics aren't known because many women never report any problems to their doctor, but it's thought that at least 50 per cent of women who have had children have some degree of prolapse.

Why me?

The main cause of prolapse is pregnancy and childbirth. Just carrying a growing baby stretches the ligaments that support the womb, and during childbirth both the pelvic-floor muscles and the tissues that support the wall of the vagina are also stretched. Not every mother gets a prolapse, but it is more likely to occur the more babies that you have, or if you have difficult prolonged labour, a large baby or a forceps delivery. Prolapse is more common in women who have had vaginal births compared to those who have given birth by caesarean.

Though many pre-menopausal women do have symptoms due to a prolapse, they become much more common after the menopause. The pelvic-floor muscles unfortunately tend to become weaker with age, though this is not inevitable – if you do regular pelvic-floor exercises you can keep them in good shape. But the lack of oestrogen means the walls of the vagina become thinner and less elastic, making them far less supportive and more likely to bulge.

Anything that increases the pressure inside a woman's abdomen can also increase the risk of developing a prolapse. Aside from pregnancy, the next biggest factor is obesity, especially those who are apple-shaped and store their excess weight around their middle. The fat doesn't just accumulate under the skin, it also collects inside the abdominal cavity and puts pressure on the organs it contains. Women who strain frequently due to constipation are also at risk of developing a prolapse, as are those with a chronic cough (yet another reason to give up smoking).

What type?

There are three main types of prolapse, depending on which pelvic organ has lost its support. They may occur in isolation, or together.

Prolapse of the front wall of the vagina is caused by either the urethra (the tube carrying urine from the bladder to the outside) or the bladder itself. A sagging urethra can cause a bulge just inside the entrance to the vagina (a urethrocele) while a sagging bladder tends to cause a large bulge slightly higher in the front vaginal wall (a cystocele). They often occur together (a cysto-urthrocele).

Prolapse at the centre of the top of the vagina is most commonly caused by the womb – a uterine prolapse. Occasionally there can be a prolapse of the space between the cervix and the back wall of the vagina, which contains loops of the small intestine. This is an enterocele.

Prolapse of the back wall of the vagina is caused by bulging of the lowest part of the bowel, the rectum. It's known as a rectocele.

Symptoms

Symptoms depend to a large extent on which organ has succumbed to gravity, and also how much it has lost its support. The most common thing that women feel, though, is that 'something is coming down'. If the cervix is halfway down the vagina, sex can be downright uncomfortable, while if the anterior or posterior walls have lost their support, you may just not feel very much at all during intercourse. Unfortunately, neither will your partner, though he may only mention this if you are in a very good, or bad, relationship. Many men don't want to say a word for fear of hurting their partner's feelings. Thankfully I have only ever had one patient who came to me, remarkably stoically, and said that her husband used the awful 'like a banana in a cathedral' phrase.

If you have a large prolapse, you may be able to feel either the front or the back wall of your vagina. Or, worse still, the cervix, bulging down through the entrance to the vagina, which can be extremely alarming, as well as uncomfortable when you sit down, and sometimes make sex nigh on impossible.

Prolapse of the bladder and urethra can make it difficult for the sphincter at the base of the bladder to work properly and can lead to stress incontinence. It can also make it difficult to empty your bladder properly, and some women find they need to change position while sitting on the loo, or use a finger to hold the vaginal wall up in order to pass urine.

Prolapse of the back wall of the vagina can make it difficult to open your bowels, and similarly needing to support the back vaginal wall with a finger in order to pass a motion. Many women say they also feel they pass more wind, or may accidentally pass wind during sex. Not exactly romantic.

So what can be done about it?

You may not need to do anything. Loads of women have a small prolapse and are either unaware of it or the symptoms that they do have really aren't bothering them at all. That said, once you know you have a prolapse, it is worth taking action to stop it getting any worse.

Top of the list is, yet again, to lose weight. I know, easier said than done, but please read Chapter 5 for more advice on this.

Try to avoid becoming constipated. This means changing your diet to include much more fibre, and making sure you drink plenty of fluids. If this doesn't do the trick, see your GP about medicines that can help. The aim should be to open your bowels every day without having to strain.

Next on the list is to do regular pelvic-floor exercises, which can help to stop a mild prolapse getting worse. Unfortunately, no exercise can re-tone, or shrink, a stretched vaginal wall. If it's bulging a lot and causing you discomfort the only way to put it right is with surgery. I'll come on to that in detail shortly.

Plastic pessaries

If you are having troublesome symptoms, and for whatever reason are keen to avoid the scalpel, a vaginal pessary may help. The ones most commonly used are ring-shaped and made of either silicone or plastic, and are placed inside the vagina. The top of the ring is up behind the cervix, and the bottom wedged behind the pubic bone. Sounds uncomfortable, but it isn't as long as the ring is the right size (which means it needs to be fitted by a doctor who has this particular skill). They can be left in place for between four and six months, then changed for a new one. I only recommend them as a long-term solution for older women who, because of other medical conditions, are not suitable for surgery, but they can be a good short-term option while you are on the waiting list, or if you are likely to want to have another baby in the near future.

Surgery

The best option for dealing with a troublesome prolapse is surgery. There are various different operations that can be performed, depending on the type and size of prolapse. These include:

- **Vaginal repair.** This involves tightening up the walls of the vagina and reinforcing the tissues behind the wall, using either strong sutures or a mesh to stop any further bulging. The operation is usually done via the vagina, so there are no cuts in the tummy wall. Either the front (an anterior repair) or back (a posterior repair) walls of the vagina can be tackled, or both, and straightforward operations can be done on a day-case basis. There is usually very little pain after an anterior repair, but there may be some discomfort to the entrance to the vagina after a posterior repair. A good surgeon will leave you with a vagina that was more like the one you had pre-babies, so most women undergoing the procedure (and their partners) are very happy with the results afterwards, though it is important to wait until everything has fully healed before 'trying it out', which is usually about six weeks.

- A **hysterectomy (removing the womb)** is often the best solution for a womb that has lost its support. In most cases the operation can be done via the vagina (again, no tummy cuts) and there is very little pain afterwards. I must stress, though, that this is not, as many women believe, done via suction – the blood vessels and ligaments supplying the womb have to be carefully cut and tied, along with the fallopian tubes. Usually the ovaries are left in place. A vaginal hysterectomy can be combined with either an anterior or vaginal repair, or both, and usually involves staying in hospital for at least a couple of days. Like a repair operation, it's perfectly possible to have sex afterwards, once everything has healed. There are some circumstances which make a vaginal hysterectomy difficult, for example, if the womb is enlarged by fibroids or if there are likely to be adhesions in the pelvis from previous surgery. In these cases, removing the womb via the abdomen may be advised.

- **An operation to hitch up the uterus or vagina.** There are various different types of operation that can be done, using either strong sutures or, more commonly, mesh, to attach the uterus to the bones of the pelvis and hold it in place. Depending on the procedure, this may involve a cut in the abdominal wall, as well as one in the vagina. These operations are usually only done when a woman is very keen not to have her womb removed.

CASE HISTORIES

Bella, age 48

HER STORY: I'm trying to lose weight, and have started doing exercise classes, but I keep accidentally wetting myself. It's so embarrassing. I always wear a pad now, but is there anything I can do to stop this happening?

MORE BACKGROUND INFORMATION: Bella's three children had all been large babies, each over 9lbs in weight, all born by normal vaginal deliveries. She had gradually put on weight since then and was aware that she needed to shed at least a stone. She admitted that though she had tried to do pelvic-floor exercises after she had her first and second babies, after number three arrived she just didn't have the time. When I examined her I found that her vaginal walls were rather slack, but the main problem was the weakness of her pelvic floor. When I asked her to cough, the walls of the lower vagina bulged downwards and she leaked a small amount of urine. The urine sample I sent off to the lab was clear, so she didn't have a urine infection.

MY ADVICE: Bella needed to do pelvic-floor exercises to tighten up the muscles that supported the base of her bladder. I gave her an instruction sheet and advised that she try to make time to do some every day. Losing weight would help, too, so despite the 'accidents' I encouraged her to keep going to her exercise classes. I warned her that the pelvic-floor exercises wouldn't work straight away, and agreed to see her again in three months' time.

Unfortunately, when we met up again, she was continuing to have problems and was still leaking on a regular basis when she did exercise. She had been making a real effort to tighten up her pelvic floor, but she didn't think it had made much difference. When I examined her there was some improvement in the tone of the muscles around the entrance to her vagina, but the walls still bulged downwards when she coughed. I suggested she needed to see a gynaecologist to discuss possible surgical treatments.

She updated me a couple of months later. The gynaecologist had suggested she have a transvaginal tape procedure, as her only problem was her lower vagina, around the base of her bladder. Other than that she didn't have a significant prolapse.

The operation was a success, she was back exercising – without leaking – a couple of weeks later.

Tanya, age 53

HER STORY: For the past few years I've been wetting myself slightly. I've been trying to work out when it's happening, but it seems a bit random. I've had episodes when I've accidentally wet myself when I've coughed or sneezed, but I've also had times when I've had to dash to the loo, and not quite made it. I always have to wear a pad, and I'm feeling a bit sore – I wonder if I've got thrush as well.

MORE BACKGROUND INFORMATION: Tanya had two children, now teenagers, with only 18 months between them. The first birth had been a long difficult labour, and she'd had a forceps delivery. She admitted she had never done pelvic-floor exercises. When I asked in more detail, she admitted she had always had a tendency to go to the loo quite frequently, as she didn't like the feeling of having a full bladder; 'I always go when I can – I've never waited until I'm desperate to go, especially now'.

When I examined her, her vagina was a little lax but that was all. Her urine sample came back clear from the lab.

MY ADVICE: It sounded as if Tanya had mixed incontinence, and I advised her that she needed urodynamic tests to sort out what was going on. She reported back that these had confirmed my diagnosis and that she had an appointment to see a specialist nurse to learn about bladder retraining, and also doing pelvic-floor exercises.

Three months on, her stress incontinence was much better but she was continuing to have to dash to the loo, and didn't have much warning when her bladder was full. She admitted that she had found the bladder retraining difficult – 'I have stopped going "just in case" whenever I can, but I'm not going to risk it if I'm travelling and don't know when I'll next be able to go, but when I'm at home I'm definitely going less often'.

I prescribed her a small dose of oxybutynin to try to relax her bladder a little, and this worked well and gave her more confidence to trust that she could 'hold on' when she was out of the house.

Paula, age 59

HER STORY: Something's not right down below. I can feel a lump in my vagina, and my husband has commented that it feels different, too – as if something is in the way when we're having sex. I'm worried it's something serious, like a tumour – that's why I'm here.

MORE BACKGROUND INFORMATION: It turned out one of the main reasons she was so worried was because she had always had a tendency to constipation, but in the last year it had got much worse, and she often had to put a finger into her vagina to help force a motion out of her back passage. She'd had two children, the first by a long difficult vaginal delivery, and the second by a caesarean. She was overweight, and was a typical apple shape, with most of her extra pounds around her middle. When I examined her genital area, I found that her womb had dropped halfway down her vagina – a uterine prolapse. The back wall of her vagina was also very lax, which meant that her rectum was bulging into her vagina – a rectocele.

MY ADVICE: I suggested to Paula that she probably needed surgery to deal with her prolapsed womb and her rectocele, but that it would also help if she tried to lose weight, and she could help her constipation problem by eating a lot more fibre.

The gynaecologist advised that she needed to have her womb removed via her vagina, and that she could have her rectocele repaired at the same time. At first she was rather alarmed by the prospect of a hysterectomy, but I explained that her womb wasn't actually doing anything any more, other than causing her discomfort. The surgery was very straightforward, and she was home a couple of days after the operation. She had quite a lot of discomfort to begin with where the repair had been done, but this improved within a week of surgery.

Lily, age 51

HER STORY: I'm forever wetting myself. Whenever I cough or I sneeze, I leak a bit. Same thing happens when I run for the bus. I wear a pad, but by the end of the day the first thing I do is have a shower to clean myself up. I thought this type of thing only happened to old ladies, and I don't classify myself as old.

MORE BACKGROUND INFORMATION: Lily had four children in her late teens and early twenties. No one had said anything to her at the time about doing pelvic-floor exercises. She admitted she was really embarrassed by her problem, which had been going on for several years, but it was only the fear of being 'smelly' that made her come and see me. Her urine sample looked cloudy, and laboratory testing confirmed that she had a urine infection. But that wasn't her only problem, as when I examined her I could see that the front wall of her vagina was very lax, and bulging downwards, and this was almost certainly causing her stress incontinence.

MY ADVICE: I gave her antibiotics, and this cleared her infection, but I also advised that she needed to see a gynaecologist to sort out her prolapse. She was advised that she needed an 'anterior repair' operation, and she only needed to stay in hospital one night for this. She is now accident – and pad-free.

SUMMARY

Problems with incontinence are actually very common among women after their mid-forties, but it's not a subject that many like to talk about, and far too many women suffer in silence, trying to cope with the problem by wearing panty liners, instead of getting medical help.

▢ There are two main forms of incontinence. Stress incontinence happens when leakage occurs on coughing, or sneezing, or during exercise. It is caused by weakness around the base of the bladder, and can often be helped by pelvic-floor exercises. Surgery to lift and support the bladder neck can be curative. Urge incontinence is caused by overactivity of the muscles found in the bladder wall, leading to a sudden need to pass urine. It can be treated with medication to relax the muscles. Some women have a combination of both types.

▢ The walls of the vagina often become lax after childbirth, but this often does not cause any symptoms until after the menopause, when lack of oestrogen makes the tissues more lax. Sagging of the front wall of the vagina can allow the bottom of the bladder to flop into the vagina, which can lead to stress incontinence. Sagging of the back vaginal wall allows the rectum (the end of the large bowel) to bulge into the vagina, leading to difficulty passing a motion.

▢ Laxity of the ligaments that support the womb can lead to it dropping downwards into the vagina. This can lead to discomfort and also difficulty with sex.

▢ All types of prolapse can be dealt with very easily with surgery.

▢ Symptoms of urine infections often change with age. Instead of causing severe stinging and pain, the only symptom may be a need to pass urine more often, and slightly offensive-smelling urine.

10

SKIN AND HAIR

Our skin and hair are perhaps our most noticeable features, and unfortunately the hormonal havoc of the menopause inevitably leads to changes in both of them.

Like all women, my complexion changed in my late forties. Having always had a bit of tendency to greasy skin, I'd always used a 'light' moisturiser, suitable for normal/combination skins. Then one day I realised this wasn't enough – within a few minutes of putting it on my face seemed parched again. Time to switch to something much richer, for 'mature, drier skin'.

Not only had the top layer of my skin changed, but along with that dryness, I realised my face had well and truly lost its youthful bloom. Lines and wrinkles had appeared, and my eyelids were beginning to droop. My lips were also looking thinner than before. I had hit middle age.

Simple ageing has a lot to do with this, but there is no doubt plunging hormone levels can play a part, too, and it's around the time of the menopause that most women, like me, realise they look older.

What I'm going to do in this chapter is start with the questions I'm most commonly asked about skin and hair. Then I'll go into more details about what happens to skin, hair and teeth, and the best way of tackling the changes that come with age. There is also a small section with some information about cosmetic procedures.

Bea, age 55

'I was dreading what the menopause would do to my appearance. I had visions of suddenly going grey and wrinkly. My hair had already started going a bit grey, but I don't think the change in my hormones made any difference to it. What did change, though, was my skin. It was much more dry, and my tendency to a bit of greasy T zone down the middle disappeared. I had to switch from using a cream for combination skin to one for dry skin. And I noticed that my skin was much more easily irritated by slightly itchy clothes. I had to stop wearing anything containing wool, or I'd be scratching at my arms within a couple of hours. I've also noticed brown marks have appeared on my hands, but that's from sun damage, not from a lack of hormones. It's a warning, though, that I've got to be much more careful about proper sun protection.'

Commonly asked questions:

My skin is much drier than it ever was before. Why is this? What do you recommend I use on this? Is it worth paying out for a really expensive cream?

It's partly due to simply growing older, but loss of oestrogen has a lot to do with it. Oestrogen helps boost natural moisture production in the skin, so dryness is common after the menopause. I'm not convinced by many of the claims on expensive creams, and I recommend using simple products designed for dry, sensitive skin. I usually recommend a cream for daytime and a serum or oil at night. You will need to be generous with the amount you use.

My skin has lost its bloom and looks dull and lifeless. Would HRT help with this?

Oestrogen helps maintain the collagen and elastin that support the skin from beneath, so after the menopause it does tend to look a bit more saggy. There is some evidence that HRT can help to maintain a more youthful appearance in the skin, but bearing in mind the side effects, you need to think long and hard whether you want to take it for this reason alone. You may also have a bit of a job convincing your doctor to prescribe it just to maintain your looks.

I've developed brown blotches on my skin, especially my hands and, worse still, a few on my face. Why is this, and what can I do about them?

These are caused by excess production of melanin, the pigment that gives fair skin a tan. They are caused by excess exposure to UV light – from either the sun or sunbeds. They can be treated with intense pulsed light (IPL) or laser, but as this is a cosmetic procedure it's not available on the NHS.

My skin used to be really quite good, but now it's a real mess. Dry on the forehead and at the sides, but red and a bit spotty on my nose and cheeks. Is this some form of acne linked to the menopause?

This sounds like rosacea. It's not linked to the change in hormones, but is common in women after the age of 40. The redness is caused by dilated tiny blood vessels in the skin, and is often much more obvious after consuming hot spicy food or alcohol. The exact reason why some women get it and others don't isn't fully understood, but it can usually be treated with metronidazole gel, or antibiotic tablets taken by mouth.

My hair seems to be much thinner and more fragile, except where I don't want it – on my upper chin! Is this due to my hormones?

Oestrogen promotes the growth of hair on the scalp, and this means that after the menopause hair does become a little thinner, and it also doesn't grow as long before falling out. Not only that, but oestrogen counteracts the effects of the small amounts of testosterone that are produced by the adrenal glands. After the menopause this testosterone becomes the dominant hormone, and this leads to an increase in growth on the face, especially above the upper lip. In later life it can also lead to thinning of the scalp hair in a 'male pattern baldness' pattern around the temples. But it is very rare for women to lose their scalp hair as dramatically as occurs in some men.

I seem to have lost a lot of my pubic hair. I've never heard this mentioned in connection with the menopause. Is it normal?

Yes. The 'sexual hair' that grows at puberty in the armpits and around the genital area is in response to the hormones produced by the ovaries. That means that at the menopause, this hair usually thins noticeably, which many women simply don't expect. There is more information about this on page 288.

My periods have stopped and my hair suddenly seems to have gone grey. Any connection?

No. This is one area where those falling oestrogen levels that occur at the menopause really don't seem to make any difference. The colour of your hair is determined by your genes and your age, not your hormone levels.

So what happens to the skin at the menopause?
Moisture and structure

Oestrogen stimulates the production of sebaceous fluid, which has a moisturising effect on the skin. So inevitably as oestrogen levels fall and the skin can become drier.

The deep structure of skin is provided by the proteins collagen and elastin, and production of these is partially controlled by oestrogen. Collagen and elastin are damaged by sunlight, and under the influence of oestrogen more is produced to repair and renew the lost tissues. But once oestrogen is lost, this 'damage limitation' process becomes much less efficient. There's more about this in the section about sunlight (page 162).

The skin, like every other organ in the body, is dependent on a good blood supply for maximum health. The growth and maintenance of the tiny blood capillaries in the skin, which supply vital blood and other nutrients, is partially controlled by oestrogen. After the menopause, there is a slight reduction in blood supply, and this contributes to a slower production of skin cells and skin thinning. This in turn means that the skin has a reduced barrier function, leading to increased water loss, dryness and general fragility.

Then there is the effect of oestrogen on the fat deposits beneath the skin. The lack of oestrogen after the menopause means fat tends to be redistributed; it is gained around the abdomen but lost from the face and neck, and also the breasts, which all tend to look less plump and sadly more droopy.

Pigmentation

The maintenance and function of melanocytes, the cells that produce the pigment melanin, is also affected. It is melanin that helps to protect the skin from damage when exposed to sunlight – a tan, which is due to increased melanin production, is nature's own protective mechanism. With less melanocytes, the skin appears slightly lighter, and when exposed to the sun tanning is less efficient, meaning the skin is likely to be more damaged. But just to be perverse, in areas of the skin that have been exposed to the UV rays over the years, melanin production may be increased, due to lack of regulation by oestrogen. This can result in brown 'age spots' appearing on sun-exposed areas, especially the face, hands and arms.

TAKING ACTION!

I'm aware that this sounds like a dreadful tale of woe, but please do not despair. Most women continue to look wonderful after the menopause. There is plenty you can do to help maintain your skin through the years of change.

Rule number one - no tanning!

Top of the list if you want to delay ageing as much as possible is to protect your skin from the sun. Some dermatologists reckon that around 80 per cent of skin ageing is due to the effects of sunlight. To get an idea of how true this is, compare the soft smooth skin of your buttocks with that on your hands and face, which will have been exposed far more to the sun.

The sun's ultraviolet light alters skin because it can penetrate through to the deep layers and damage collagen, the protein that provides skin with its elasticity. This in itself can make skin look more lined and wrinkled, even before the menopause.

Some people's skins are naturally better protected from the sun because their skin contains more melanin, the natural dark pigment that helps prevent UV light penetrating the deeper layers. This is why dark-skinned women tend to look younger than white-skinned women of the same age – they are naturally better protected from the sun.

The more you can hide your skin from the damaging UV rays in sunlight, the more you will slow down the ageing process. This means steering clear of sunbeds as well as sunshine – the UV from sunbeds is very ageing. Everyone needs a little exposure to sunshine to stimulate vitamin D production in their skin, but this can be done early or late in the day when the sun is less strong, from your arms and legs. Your face and your hands, the bits that have almost certainly been exposed to too much sun in the past, do not have to be involved in vitamin D production. They should always be protected.

Rule number two - no smoking

After sunshine, the most important influence on your skin is smoking. You only have to look at a picture of a woman who has smoked all her life to see how the habit has left her with fine lines, especially around the mouth, and dull, lifeless skin. This is because smoking causes narrowing of all arteries, including the tiny capillaries in the skin, starving the cells of oxygen and nutrients. Though this damage is sadly irreversible, it's never too late to stop it getting worse by giving up. It will not only help protect your skin but will also have major benefits for your health overall.

Rule number three - moisturise!

Even if you have felt you have never needed to use a moisturiser before, once you lose your oestrogen your complexion needs some outside help to stop it looking – and feeling – a bit like a dried prune. But this does not need to cost you a fortune; some of the best creams come very cheaply and can be bought along with your groceries at your local supermarket.

So which product?

There is a vast array of face creams available, varying in price between a few pence and several hundred pounds per small pot. Many of the more expensive ones in particular make claims that applying their magic potion will take years off your appearance, and cosmetic companies are endlessly coming up with new ingredients which, they hint, will make us look young again. Vitamins A, C and E, green tea and scientific-sounding chemicals such as CoQ10, neuropeptides and phosphatidylcholine are now turning up in products, along with collagen. It's easy to think that a cream that is labelled as a 'cosmeceutical', or is marketed by a dermatologist is going to be better than something that's simply labelled as a moisturiser. However, by law cosmetics are not allowed to alter the structure of the skin. If they made such a major difference, they would be classified as drugs, and their manufacturers would be forced to carry out expensive tests to prove their products were safe and effective.

Beauty experts spend their life trying out different creams, and there is no doubt that some do seem to be better than others. But as always, it's a matter of individual choice, and what your best friend swears by may be no good for you. Don't be fooled by a high price tag and fancy packaging. Frequent applications of something cheap and cheerful can work wonders for most women. My main recommendation for older women is to be careful about added perfume – at the menopause a skin that previously could take anything that was slapped on it may suddenly become sensitive. But beware the labels 'dermatologically tested' or 'hypo-allergenic'. They sound very scientific, but are pretty meaningless, as there is no medical definition or formal legal certification requirement for either term. I've seen some awful allergic reactions to 'hypo-allergenic' products. Better to look for a basic product that says it is 'fragrance free' and suitable for sensitive skins. If you find yourself reacting to lots of creams, start reading the fine print and the list of ingredients to see if you can identify a common culprit. Unfortunately, many standard preservatives used in creams and lotions can be allergenic. If the problem persists, see your GP, and see if you would benefit from formal allergy testing.

What about exfoliating and peeling?

Exfoliating aims to remove some of the top layer of cells of the skin to reveal the younger ones beneath, making your skin look and feel smoother and softer, using a physical process with tiny grains in a cream – a bit like using a gentle Brillo pad. This process won't actually remove wrinkles but it can help a moisturising cream to penetrate a little deeper through the surface of the skin, which can make it look plumper. However, it needs to be done with caution on a more sensitive, post-menopausal skin, which can easily become red and flaky from overenthusiastic or frequent exfoliation.

Peels take the process a little further. These aim to remove the outer surface of the skin using chemicals, usually a mild acid. There is some evidence that this can increase the rate at which the skin renews itself, and therefore make it look plumper and less wrinkled. However, again there is the risk that it can make your face really sore, and ironically this is most likely to happen to fair-skinned people whose skin naturally tends to age more quickly than others.

And retinoids? I keep reading about them.

There is some good evidence that tretinoin, a chemical related to vitamin A, can help boost collagen production and help the appearance of skin that has been damaged by the sun. However, it's really powerful stuff that can make the skin dry and irritated, and very sensitive to damage from the sun. Tretinoin can also be teratogenic, with the potential to alter the development of a boy in the womb, so they are only available on prescription. Products containing tretinoin need to be used with extreme care on older skins. Retinol, which is the scientific term for vitamin A, is very different. It is much milder than tretinoin – so mild, in fact, that it is questionable whether it really makes any difference to the skin. It is available in face creams you can buy over the counter.

No matter what you slap on your face, by far the most important two things you can do to maintain your complexion are to protect your face from the sun, and to stop smoking. Nothing else comes close, and there is no point in spending a small fortune on skincare products if you tan your face at the first opportunity every summer.

Sunscreens

All women, of all ages, should apply a broad spectrum sunscreen every morning. Make it part of your routine, like cleaning your teeth. This becomes especially important once you are in your forties, and the chances are you've already exposed your face to far too much sun. It should provide protection against both UVA and UVB rays. UVB rays are the ones that burn, and are also the main rays that increase the risk of skin cancer, including melanoma, while UVA rays are the ones that penetrate deep into the dermis and cause ageing.

The protection against UVB is marked with the SPF factor, which is an indication of how much longer you can stay out in the sun without burning compared to having no protection. So an SPF of 15 theoretically allows you stay out 15 times longer, and SPF 30, 30 times longer. The higher the SPF, the more you will pay for the product, and even though some creams and lotions claim they provide all-day protection, I still recommend frequent application rather than relying on just one.

UVA protection is marked with stars, and for good protection you need a product that has four or five stars. A statement on the label 'provides UVA protection' with no indication of the amount is not good enough!

There is also some research that indicates that the infra-red part of the sun's ultraviolet rays can contribute to skin damage, and some products now provide additional protection against damaging infra-red rays. As more evidence about this emerges, no doubt more products will provide this, too.

So which product?

Some dermatologists favour sunscreens based on 'physical' agents, such as titanium dioxide and zinc oxide, which sit on the skin and prevent the sun's rays getting to the collagen below. They are the ones you see on sportsmen with white streaks on the nose and lips, and it is true they can be more difficult to rub in than other sunscreens. They are also less likely to cause allergic reactions than those containing chemical sunscreens. Chemical sunscreens, which are by far the more widely available, contain ingredients with long, unpronounceable names that penetrate the skin and block the damaging effects of the sun's rays, and usually can be applied with no noticeable residue. At night, there is no need to cover your face with suncream, but even if you've never done it before, the increased tendency to dryness after the menopause makes applying a moisturiser a common-sense move. It will help your skin look less parched and, perhaps more importantly, feel more comfortable, too.

Eyes

It is also important to protect your eyes as well as your complexion. UV light is the main cause of cataracts and can also damage the retina, the light-sensitive membrane at the back of the eye. Invest in good sunglasses that have confirmed UV protection – which means checking they have an EU certification mark. Buy them from a reputable retailer, ideally an optician, to avoid being duped by fakes.

ROSACEA

There isn't room in this book to delve into every different skin condition that can affect menopausal women, but I think rosacea deserves a mention. This is a skin condition that commonly starts rearing its head in the early forties, and often continues – and may become worse – during and after the menopause.

Symptoms include pustules and spots that can look like acne, along with flushing and facial redness. The cheeks are often the worst affected, and the redness especially is worse after eating a spicy meal, drinking alcohol or exposure to the sun. Occasionally the eyes are affected, too, causing dryness, a gritty feeling and inflammation of the eyelids (blepharitis).

The condition can occur in men, too, but it's far more common in women. The cause isn't known but it may be linked to an abnormal immune reaction in the skin, leading to inflammation. It is also thought that a tiny mite called *Demodex folliculorum* may be involved. It lives harmlessly on the skin of many people, but higher numbers are found in those with rosacea. Damage to the tiny capillaries in the skin from the sun may also play a role.

Unfortunately, there is no cure for rosacea, but the condition can usually be controlled with either a gel containing the antimicrobial metronidazole, or with tetracycline antibiotics taken by mouth. Many months of treatment are usually required before there is a really noticeable improvement, though. Treatment may need to be continued intermittently for years. It is also important to always use a sunblock, and foundations with a green tinge (yes, they do exist!) can be very helpful for toning down the redness.

COSMETIC PROCEDURES

It's around the time of the menopause that many women start to seriously think about having 'a little work' done on their face or their body.

We've all seen pictures of celebrities who look younger with each passing year. Airbrushing means that lines and wrinkles often disappear from published images, especially in the pages of glossy magazines. Or we see a friend who somehow looks more youthful than before, and we think, 'well, if she looks that good, then so can I'.

We live in a youth-orientated age – though thankfully I think this is beginning to change, just a bit – and while some women are prepared to grow and look old, gracefully or not, many will go to extreme lengths to take away the evidence of the passing years.

Cosmetic procedures – be it fillers, Botox or going under the knife – are now big business, and so readily available that you can pop out in your lunch break and come back a different-looking woman.

Though many have undoubtedly felt they looked more attractive after having 'work', the fact is that in the UK this is a very poorly regulated industry and cosmetic procedures can, and do, go wrong and it's far more difficult to rectify than a colouring disaster at the hairdresser's.

The last thing I want to be is judgemental about whether you opt to have a filler, or something more. That is very much for each individual woman to decide, and there is no doubt that removing lines and wrinkles, or drooping eyelids, can make a huge difference to self-confidence and self-esteem in many women. But what I am really passionate about is that it should be done safely, by someone who is properly qualified, that you understand the risks involved, and that you know exactly who will help – and at what cost – if things go wrong.

Dermal fillers

These aim to fill out lines and wrinkles and make lips or sunken scars appear fuller. There are many different types, and effects usually last between four and nine months. The more that is put in, the greater the effect and the longer it will last – which is bad news if you end up resembling a trout. Side effects can include infection at the injection site, lumpiness and scarring, and there have been reports of filler inserted near the eyes migrating to block the retinal artery, causing blindness (though this is very rare).

Fillers are currently inserted by all sorts of people, including dentists and nurses as well as doctors. There is no established qualification required, and though you may think that a doctor would be best, a really skilled nurse could be as good as anyone else.

Botox

This is the common abbreviation for botulinum toxin, which blocks nerve impulses, which in turns paralyses and relaxes muscles. Many wrinkles are caused by contractions of the underlying muscles, and Botox can smooth these out. It takes effect three to seven days after the injection and lasts three to six months. With repeated treatments, the effect may last longer. Botox can unfortunately result in facial muscles that don't move at all, giving the face a mask-like appearance. Other possible side effects include double vision and the drooping of a lid or eyebrow. Botox is a prescription-only medicine, and in theory should only be injected by a doctor or a well-trained nurse working under a doctor's supervision. Unfortunately, in some clinics, the doctor writes the prescription then it's administered by someone far less qualified.

Lasers

Lasers work by destroying the surface tissue, which then repairs itself with new cells. Lasers can be used to remove acne scars, birthmarks, sun damage and wrinkles. Different types of laser can penetrate the skin to different depths and the skin, which initially takes up to 10 days to heal, can look red for several weeks afterwards. Lasers can be dangerous and cause burning and damage the eyes. All clinics offering laser treatment have to be registered, and though it's best done by an experienced doctor or nurse, some beauty therapists can now use low-powered lasers.

Surgical procedures

These include face lifts, liposuction or breast enlargement or reduction, and should, by law, only be carried out in hospitals or clinics registered and regularly inspected by the Care Quality Commission (and the results are available on their website). The doctor doing the procedure – and you should know who he or she is – should not only be fully medically qualified, but have a higher surgical qualification, preferably an FRCS Plast, which means they have undergone training and passed an exam in plastic surgery. Ideally they should also be a member of the British Association of Aesthetic Plastic Surgeons. You will pay more for a person with these confirmed skills, but getting a cut-price deal with someone less qualified could cost you dearly in terms of a poor result.

My recommendations

- You should never undertake any sort of cosmetic procedure on the spur of the moment. You should think long and hard about it and ask yourself why you want to have it done. Changing your appearance may not be the best way of improving your relationship, or your self-esteem.

● Be realistic about what can be achieved; generally this is a field where 'less is more' and trying to look twenty years younger is likely to backfire. Just looking less tired can be a far better aim.

● Do a lot of homework about the procedure itself, the place where you intend to have it done and especially the person wielding the needle or the knife. It's not good enough if a clinic says 'it's one of the staff'.

● Make sure you speak to your actual surgeon beforehand, and check their qualifications and experience. Many clinics offering dermal fillers and Botox go unchecked, with no inspections of either care standards or staff qualifications.

● Be especially wary of a hard sell if you go into a clinic and make enquiries – a good clinic will willingly give you information and offer you time to think about it.

HAIR

Our hair, like everything else, changes with age, and can be affected by hormones – just think of what happens during pregnancy, when hair becomes thick and lush, only to start thinning dramatically a few months after the baby is born.

The natural hair cycle

Hair growth goes through a natural cycle. The first part, the anagen phase, is the growth phase, and lasts an average of three to five years. Hair grows from a follicle on average around half an inch a month, so if left to grow a hair can ultimately reach between 18 and 30 inches. Next comes a short catagen, or transitional phase, that only lasts about two weeks, during which there is a slight change to the blood supply to the hair follicle, from where the hair grows. Finally, there is the telogen phase, when the hair follicle rests, then falls out. This phase lasts anything from one to four months. Then within two weeks a new anagen phase starts from the follicle. Ten to fifteen per cent of the hairs on the head are normally in this phase at any one time. The average woman has between 100,000 and 150,000 hairs on her head, so this means it's normal to lose on average about 100 hairs a day.

Oestrogen helps to keep follicles in the anagen phase, which is why during pregnancy, when oestrogen levels are high, many women notice that their hair becomes much thicker. Far fewer follicles enter the telogen phase, so fewer hairs fall out.

So what happens at the menopause?

At the menopause, the falling oestrogen levels mean the growing phase becomes shorter, with the result being that hair cannot grow as long as it used to before falling out.

And what about pubic hair?

Low oestrogen levels also have an effect on what is termed 'secondary sexual hair' – the hair that grows at puberty in the armpits and pubic area. This hair does not grow so fast, and can noticeably thin – which is good news if you were always prone to hairy armpits. However, many women are shocked by the change in their pubic hair, which may become much more sparse than before. Sadly, this is rarely talked about, and I do have women coming to see me in the surgery about it, worried there is something seriously wrong. It can also, of course, have an effect on how 'sexually attractive' you may feel, but to a lesser extent, it happens to men as well, and a mature older partner should be understanding – and after all, there is way more to being attractive than a hefty bush.

And then there is testosterone ...

Before the menopause, oestrogen has a balancing effect on the testosterone produced by the ovaries and also the adrenal glands. After the menopause, testosterone becomes the dominant hormone affecting hair. It can reduce the thickness of each hair shaft, resulting in generally thinner hair. Not only this, but it can promote hair loss in a 'male pattern balding' pattern, with hair loss around the temples and crown. This effect is usually very slow, though, and often only becomes noticeable in later old age.

But there is another effect of that dominant testosterone. As in men, testosterone can promote the growth of facial hair, especially along the upper lip. Before the menopause, this is kept in check by oestrogen, but after the change you may well notice the growth of a moustache. The savings you make waxing your intimate area need to be spent on your face instead.

What about other things? What about my diet?

Though changing hormones can affect hair, there are other factors that can have a dramatic effect on hair growth, and if your crowning glory is not what it was, these shouldn't be forgotten.

Growth of hair requires the right nutrients, and crash dieting or semi-starving yourself in an attempt to keep your figure can result in quite marked hair loss. Hair growth also requires micronutrients, especially iron and zinc. Many women have suboptimal levels, especially of iron, due to a combination of blood loss through periods and eating little red meat. Though blood loss stops at the menopause, unless you make up the deficit, levels will stay low. The lower limit of a 'normal' iron level is 20mmol/L, but experts reckon that a level of 50 or more is required for optimum hair growth. Zinc deficiency is less common, but it's worth having it checked.

Thinning, dry hair can also be a sign of an underactive thyroid, and hair loss may also occur after a serious illness, because of changes to levels of nutrients to the hair follicle.

My advice for tackling thinning hair

- Check what you are eating to make sure you are giving your hair the nutrients it needs. Protein is especially important, and if you are watching your weight you may not be getting enough. The average woman needs about 45 grams of protein a day.

- Treat your hair gently. After the menopause it is more fragile than before. Don't drag a brush through it after washing it, or when it's tangled. Get a special wide-toothed comb – they are cheap.

- Switch to a conditioner for dry hair and give it the time to let it work. This means leaving it on for at least five minutes (preferably a lot longer) at least once a fortnight, covered with a thin plastic bath hat. If you are like me and wash your hair in a shower, this can be a real challenge, but I've learnt that it really can make a difference.

- Minoxidil lotion can help stimulate hair growth. It has been a popular remedy for men with male pattern baldness for many years, and a formulation is available for women of all ages. Sadly, it's not a permanent solution – hair will revert to how nature intended once its use has stopped. It's not available on the NHS, and it's not cheap, but if you are having a hair crisis I reckon it's a better way to treat yourself than spending a fortune on expensive shampoos.

But I've got completely bald patches. Is that the menopause?

No. It's more likely to be alopecia areata. This is an altogether different condition from age- and menopause-related hair thinning. Completely bald patches appear, and the scalp appears smooth, with no hair growth at all. It may affect just a small area, or at its worst the whole head, and the eyebrows and eyelashes may fall out, too. It's thought to be an autoimmune problem, with the body's own immune system reacting against the hair follicles. It is more common in those who have other autoimmune conditions, particularly affecting the thyroid. In many it is thankfully a temporary condition but in some it may last for years. Treatment is difficult and best supervised by a specialist. Local application of strong steroid cream may help; if not oral steroids or stronger immune-modulator drugs by mouth, with the aim of dampening down the abnormal immune reaction.

Going grey

By the time you hit the menopause, the chances are you will have a fair smattering of grey hairs. The age at which greying starts appears to be almost entirely due to genetics – if one or more of your parents started going grey in their twenties then the chances are you will, too. And of course there are other lucky ones who maintain their hair colour into their eighties or nineties. But on average the '50' rule applies – by the age of 50, 50 per cent of people will have 50 per cent grey hair. And this is one where actually the menopause doesn't seem to make any difference.

As yet there are no special diets, supplements, vitamins or proteins that have been proven to slow or in any way affect the greying process, although you'll find many products claiming to do this. If you don't want to go grey, you're far better spending your money on a good, gentle hair colour than trying to take something by mouth.

A WORD ABOUT TEETH

A lot of women have asked me about the effect of menopause on their teeth, as it's about this time of life that they notice their teeth look different.

Teeth, like every other part of the body, alter with age, and given all the biting and chewing they have to do, it's not surprising. But losing your teeth should not be part of ageing – if looked after well your teeth should last a lifetime. That said, the surface enamel does inevitably become worn, and the dentin, the layer in the middle of each tooth, becomes thicker and darker. Together, this gives the appearance of less white, more yellow teeth. The wearing of the enamel also means slight gaps appear between the teeth, and to clean between the teeth properly you'll probably find you need to use small interdental brushes instead of a length of floss.

Not only this, but the gums slowly recede, exposing more of the base of the tooth – hence the expression 'becoming long in the tooth'. If the roots become exposed, teeth will be more sensitive. The jaw bones also shrink, and this can be marked in women with osteopenia and particularly osteoporosis, leading to slight loosening of the teeth.

Of course, a set of slightly yellow gnashers isn't exactly a good look and can be ageing. Not only that, but NHS dental services have been so drastically cut that having anything other than a straightforward filling can be hideously expensive. So an important part of looking after yourself after the menopause is to really spend time looking after your teeth.

That means:

- Cleaning all five surfaces of every tooth twice a day, not just the top and the inner and outer surfaces. The place where teeth are most likely to develop caries is on the surface adjacent to the next tooth, which is of course the most fiddly bit to clean. But clean you must, using an interdental brush near the gums, and floss where the teeth touch at the top.

- Get an electric toothbrush. They really are better than manual ones.

- Making sure you get all the plaque off your teeth, especially near the gums. Plaque is a combination of food debris and bacteria, and if not removed it causes inflammation of the gums. This in turn causes 'pockets' next to the tooth, where yet more gunk collects. Your gums will bleed, you'll have bad breath, and your teeth may become loose and fall out. Not only that, but there is now a link between inflamed gums and heart disease – it seems the chemicals linked with the inflammation affect the coronary arteries that supply the heart as well.

● Avoid acidic foods and drinks, as these can dissolve the enamel. Fruit juices are an obvious culprit, but so is anything fizzy, including water – those bubbles come from carbonic acid. If you do have something acidic, don't clean your teeth straight away afterwards – you'll just brush away the softened enamel. Instead, give your saliva, which is very alkaline, at least half an hour to neutralise the acid.

● See your dentist for regular check-ups and a hygienist at least twice a year for a really thorough clean.

What about teeth whitening?

One of the best ways of making yourself look a little younger is to make your teeth look less yellow and more white and pearly. There are lots of toothpastes available that claim to whiten your teeth, but by law they only contain very weak whitening ingredients. The only way to effectively whiten your teeth is to use products that are much stronger, and only available from a qualified dentist. This is for a good reason – the strength of bleach they contain can irritate your gums and make your teeth very sensitive, and it is essential you have a full dental check-up before you embark on using them. Be realistic, though – you only want to go a few shades less yellow – do not try to aim for very pearly Hollywood-style white teeth that everyone notices before anything else!

SUMMARY

📖 The loss of oestrogen that occurs at the menopause usually makes the skin much more dry. Even if you have never done so, now is the time when using a moisturiser should become as much an everyday essential as cleaning your teeth.

📖 Dry skin is also more prone to irritation from perfumes and other chemicals, such as biological detergents, and also from slightly itchy fabrics. You may find it impossible to wear wool next to your skin, especially around your neck.

📖 Hormone changes also mean that the skin loses some of its deep support, making it a little more saggy and more prone to lines and wrinkles.

📖 Though the skin inevitably changes with age, far more damage is done by sunlight and smoking. Though there is nothing you can do about past exposure, protecting your face from UV light and stopping smoking are essential for preserving your complexion.

📖 Hair also becomes a little thinner after the menopause, and does not grow as long. It is also more fragile, so needs to be treated gently.

📖 Secondary sexual hair – in the armpits and groin – can become much more sparse.

📖 If you decide to have any cosmetic work done, think about it carefully and do a lot of research beforehand, especially investigating the experience of the practitioner or surgeon.

11

THE OTHER SIDE
– LIFE AFTER THE
MENOPAUSE

Rose, age 58

'I really wasn't looking forward to the menopause. I had in my head that it meant I was getting old, that my youth had gone and that I'd have to endure years of flushes and sweats. In fact, I didn't have too bad a time of it when my periods stopped, and the few sweats that I did have had gone six months later. What happened was that I wasn't irritable for a week each month, and I felt somehow calmer, on more of an even keel. I'm able to concentrate at work better, and am much more productive. I've looked after my skin, waiting for wrinkles to appear, but they haven't. I don't think my appearance has changed much at all really. I reckon I aged much more quickly when I was trying to juggle mothering two young kids and working four days a week. Yes, my skin is more dry, and I have to allow time to moisturise not just my face but my arms and my legs every morning, but I don't reckon that is much of a hardship.

If I look back at the last 10 years, the worst thing for me, emotionally, was when my eldest went off to university, and that happened well before the menopause. I howled into my pillow – I couldn't believe my little baby had gone. Of course, he was back in the holidays, and that semi-transition helped no end when he did finally leave to be in his own flat. Both my children are living away from home now, and in many ways my life has now reverted to how it was in my twenties, but without all the traumas that went with being that age. I'm settled in a good relationship, and now that my biological clock has finally stopped, I have a new sense of freedom, I can work long hours without feeling guilty, and can spend my spare time on myself. The menopause just meant no more periods, that's all.'

Harriet, age 55

'Everything I read about the menopause sounded awful. Flushes, sweats, dreadful periods, mood swings, depression. And afterwards, well I'd be joining the ranks of the well and truly middle-aged, wouldn't I? That I'd be "too old" for promotion at work, that I'd be planning for my retirement. Not exactly something to look forward to.

The reality has been so different. Yes, I did have a few horrendous days of heavy bleeding, and my body thermostat went off kilter for a few months, but I could cope. I reckon the whole process took nine months, max. And then I realised I wasn't having to take my cardigan on and off, and that I was actually sleeping better than I had for years. And I was more relaxed about sex, because I wasn't worried about accidentally getting pregnant any more.

In retrospect, no one at work had a clue that I'd gone through the change, and in fact I've been promoted in the last year and taken on a lot more responsibility. Yes, I'm topping up my pension as much as I can, but that's only sensible now that I'm in my fifties. I'm not planning on retiring for years.

But being honest, even though I feel and look very well, the menopause has made me realise my body isn't as young as it used to be, and I am taking a bit more care of myself than I used to. I try to exercise regularly, as I think that's very important, and I'm trying to watch what I eat and shed some of the extra weight I've been carrying for far too long. I was invited recently for an NHS health check at my surgery, and I'm going to make sure I go – I reckon a few years ago I wouldn't have bothered.'

Christine, age 59

'Even I find it difficult to believe, but I reckon that at nearly 60 I'm having the best time of my life. I'm still working, but I'm not trying to climb the greasy career pole any more – I'm in a fairly senior position, so I'm just making sure I do my job properly and responsibly. I also like mentoring younger people. I have made it a rule not to work at weekends any more, and I make sure I take my full holiday entitlement. I have three grandchildren, and I love seeing them, and will do babysitting duty at weekends, but only when it suits me. I don't think I'm being selfish – I've worked hard all my life, and this is *my* time now. I'm keeping my mind and body active – I'm learning Spanish, which I've always wanted to do, and play tennis every weekend, and I also go on long bike rides and hikes. I'm still able to wear stylish clothes and I want to look trendy, but in an age-appropriate way. I'm definitely calmer and more confident, and more at ease with who I am than I was when I was younger.'

The aim of this book is to help you understand, and cope with, what can be a huge physical and mental upheaval in your life. Hopefully you will now be armed with enough information to cope, just a little bit better, with what can be the unpleasant and undignified events that occur at the menopause.

After 50 years on the planet, you are inevitably older, but also much wiser. And what I really want to emphasise is life does not end with the menopause. For many women, the freedom from having to cope with monthly mood swings, bleeding and pain, and not having to worry about accidentally becoming pregnant, is really welcome.

And let's get things in perspective. The average life expectancy of a woman in the UK is now 83 years, and getting longer. With oestrogen production starting between age 10 and 11, and the menopause at 50, that means that a woman has oestrogen for a little less than half her life.

Yes, feeling and looking good after the menopause can take a little more effort, and the words 'high maintenance' take on a whole new meaning. But we all know older women, from their fifties onwards, who not only look fabulous but are reaching the peaks of their careers, or taking on new roles, and clearly are happy and fulfilled.

However, though many do have excellent health, this is a time when you shouldn't take your body for granted, and looking after yourself should be a priority.

Oestrogen helps to protect your body from heart disease, and that means that sadly the risk of heart attacks and strokes rapidly rises after the age of 50. But this is not inevitable – you can keep your risk of heart disease low if you adjust your diet and lifestyle to compensate for the lack of oestrogen.

That means:

- Taking regular exercise. This should be the number one priority for everyone. If you could put the benefits of exercise into a bottle it would be a wonder drug. Apart from helping to keep your weight down, it can help to maintain your muscles, keep you strong and fit, and help prevent heart disease, strokes and osteoporosis. Just because you are over 50 does not mean you can't take up a new sport, or take one that you are doing already to a more challenging level. I'm aiming to do my first triathlon next year!

- Watching your diet. Keeping your weight down is more difficult now because your metabolism will have slowed down, but it's quite possible if you are careful with what you are eating, and your portion sizes. Especially avoid foods high in saturated fat, which are not only laden with calories but also will raise your blood cholesterol levels. Be firm with yourself and step on the scales twice a month, and take action if you see the reading moving in the wrong direction.

- Be breast aware. The risk of breast cancer rises with age, and at the age of 50, one in 43 women will develop invasive breast cancer in the next 10 years. So make sure you know what your breasts feel like, by checking them once every fortnight or so. That way, you're likely to spot something unusual early.

- Be 'bone aware'. Make sure you eat enough calcium and get enough vitamin D. If you think you may be at increased risk of osteoporosis, speak to your doctor.

- Look at your stools. It's amazing how many people never do this. Like your breasts, learn what is normal for you, and if that changes, get medical advice. Like most cancer, the risk of bowel cancer rises with age, and the first sign is often a change in your bowel habit – harder, smaller stools, or stools streaked with blood.

- Try to find out if there are any diseases that appear to run in your family. If there have been several cases of cancer, or heart disease, speak to your doctor to see if you should have any special screening tests.

- Looking after your skin and checking it for marks or bumps that are itchy, changing colour, growing or bleeding. Get someone else to check your back.

- Don't ignore any unusual symptoms. You are now at an age where a persistent cough, a change in your bowel habit, pain or discomfort anywhere, abnormal bleeding or unexplained weight loss should trigger a trip to your doctor.

MENTAL HEALTH

Anyone, of any age, can be affected by mental health issues. Though it's true that mood swings, anxiety and depression are more common when your hormones are in a state of flux around the time of the menopause, depression and anxiety can, and often do, affect women in their fifties and sixties. Life events can often be a trigger – such as an elderly parent becoming ill or dying, or children leaving home. It can be very difficult to adjust to having an empty nest, and it may become apparent that children were the glue that was holding together an otherwise broken relationship.

Looking after your mental health is every bit as important as caring for your physical health. That means:

- Aiming for a good work–life balance. I am all too aware that I get tired much more easily than I did in my twenties, and if I work a 12-hour day I am exhausted. If I am tired or stressed I get irritable, and I also tend to have that extra glass of wine. Making time for sleep and relaxation is always important, but especially so once you are over 50. Though hopefully you still have a good life ahead of you, you never know what is round the corner. Your career may be important and fulfilling now, but at this age you should not be working all hours at the expense of having time for your family, yourself, or hobbies.

- Making time for yourself, and doing the things *you* want to do. This is not being selfish; at this time of life, it is being sensible.

- Recognising when you are tired, or taking on too much, and learning to slow down and, most importantly, to say 'no'. I see far too many women in their fifties who are running themselves ragged trying to combine their jobs with looking after elderly parents who live miles away, cooking and doing the washing for adult offspring who live at home because they can't afford to pay rent, and then take on a voluntary role in the local community because it would have seemed bad not to. Sound familiar?

- If you feel that you are not coping, or are feeling low or anxious, seek help. There is nothing wrong with this; it is not a sign of weakness. The day of the 'stiff upper lip' should now be well gone. And as with so many health issues, mental problems are always easier to tackle if addressed early on.

HEALTH MOT

Nearly all diseases are easy to tackle if caught early. Your body is like a car – as it grows older it's liable to develop faults, so just like a car, a woman of 50-plus should have a regular health MOT, even if you feel perfectly fit and well.

This should include:

- At least every three years, a mammogram. This is offered on the NHS. The incidence of breast cancer rises with age, and just because no one in your family has been affected does not mean that you are immune.

- Every five years – a cervical smear test. Ask if you can have a pelvic check at the same time, for swelling of the ovaries or womb. If you've never had an abnormal smear, there is no need to have smear tests after the age of 65.

- Every two years – a blood pressure check along with a check of your blood cholesterol level. If you are fond of a drink, have your liver function checked as well. Women are more at risk of alcohol-induced liver damage than men. If you are afraid of having this done, ask yourself why!

- Every three years – a blood glucose test. Diabetes becomes more common with increasing age, and the symptoms can be so vague you may think you are just tired.

- Every two years – an eye test. By now your eyesight will be changing and you'll probably need glasses. A good eye test will also be able to detect signs of other diseases, such as high blood pressure and diabetes.

EPILOGUE

Many women dread the thought of the menopause, and what it might bring. Though some women sail through it, and the only change they notice is that they are not having periods anymore, they are sadly in the minority. For many women, the menopause is a time of huge physical and emotional change.

Hopefully this book will have given you the information to understand what is happening to your body, and why, and most importantly, the knowledge of how best to deal with the upheaval that nature has thrown at you.

Apart from dealing with unwelcome symptoms such as flushes, sweats and mood swings, the menopause marks a time when silent changes inside your body mean that having health check-ups becomes really important. You may never have paid any attention to your bones before, but now is the time to find out if you are risk of osteoporosis. Similarly the rise in cholesterol levels after the menopause means that heart disease can, and sometimes does, become much more of a reality. As always, taking action early really can give you the best chance of giving yourself a long, health life.

Nutrition also becomes increasingly important. The menopause marks a time when many women suddenly realise they are piling on weight for no apparent reason. But this does not have to be an inevitable part of being post menopausal. If you keep an eye on your food intake, adjust your calorie intake, and above all, stay active, you can keep middle-age spread at bay. And once you are past the worst, you really can look forward to a period of stability your physical and mental state. Indeed many women in their 'third age' experience a positive rejuvenation in both their mind and body. I hope you are one of them!

INDEX